PRACTICAL BAZAAR MEDICINES

PRACTICAL BAZAAR MEDICINES

WITH OVER
200 USEFUL PRESCRIPTIONS

G. T. BIRDWOOD

GYAN

Published by

Gyan Publishing House
5, Ansari Road
Daryaganj, New Delhi-110002
Phone: 011-47034999, 9811692060
E-mail: books@gyanbooks.com

Distribution Network
gyanbooks.com
India, USA, Canada, UK, Australia, France

ISBN : 978-81-212-3913-4 (PB)
First Published, 1936

2nd Impression 2020

Printed at: Gyan Press, Delhi.

Practical Bazaar Medicines
Author: G. T. Birdwood

PREFACE TO THIRD EDITION.

THERE is still a steady demand for this practical little book. A new edition is now needed. The object of the book is kept firmly in view, namely to supply a handy list of practical bazaar medicines and a list of useful prescriptions made up from them. Several new prescriptions have been added.

The bazaar medicines pharmacopœia given in Chapter III shows what a large range of usefulness bazaar medicines have. Very many good prescriptions for relief of indigestion, flatulence, constipation, fever, influenza, scurvy and other symptoms and diseases as well as many good bitter tonics will be found in it.

I have also added a Chapter IV on stock medicines needed for emergencies and first aid which some may find useful.

1936. G. T. BIRDWOOD.

PREFACE TO FIRST EDITION.

THIS small book on Bazaar Medicines is written with the hope that it may be useful to medical men working in Indian districts, as those in medical charge of Branch District Dispensaries, Mission Dispensaries and those in private practice far away from chemist shops.

It is of a very simple and practical nature and puts forward a number of definite prescriptions which can be made up from bazaar medicines.

The brief list of bazaar medicines, according to their actions given in Chapter I, will show what a large range of practical therapeutics bazaar medicines cover. If a medical man has a good knowledge of these, he can treat many minor maladies and relieve much suffering at a very little cost.

It must be remembered that a great many of the maladies of everyday life, for which doctors are consulted and for which people come as out-patients to dispensaries, are of a minor nature, as coughs, colds, indigestion, ulcers, sore eyes, sore throats, worms. Bazaar medicines intelligently used have a sufficiently practical and wide enough range to meet most of these maladies.

There is no question that bazaar medicines are much cheaper. A bottle of European medicine costs As. 8 to Rs. 2, while a bazaar medicine costs a few pice. District Board Dispensaries can give a vast amount of medical relief at very little cost if bazaar medicines are intelligently and largely used. Even in such epidemics as influenza, plague, cholera and relapsing fever, bazaar drugs can give much relief.

At the big medical schools, attached to our big hospitals, in the course on Materia Medica, Indian plants and drugs receive attention, but in the wards of the big hospitals, which institutions have an ample supply of European drugs, bazaar medicines are practically never prescribed, so that men leave the medical schools with little practical knowledge of prescribing bazaar medicines.

Also the books on Indian medicinal plants and drugs by Nadkarni, Khory, Mooden Sherrif and Chopra, interesting and useful as they are, give a vast amount of detail and describe many drugs which are practically never used. Nadkarni describes 419 drugs. Many are of great value, many have very slight therapeutic value. The majority are of no practical value to the medical practitioner. Big manufacturing and pharmaceutical chemists are needed in India, who can make and standardize preparations and put them on the market.

It is hoped this little book, by being very brief and putting up definite prescriptions of bazaar drugs, may be of help to practitioners. It is interleaved with blank pages, so that practitioners can add useful prescriptions of their own to those already given.

CONTENTS.

CHAPTER I.

LIST OF THE MOST USEFUL AND PRACTICAL BAZAAR MEDICINES ACCORDING TO THEIR ACTIONS.

This short list will show what a large range of therapeutics can be covered by bazaar medicines.

Alteratives.

	PAGE.
AMMONIUM CHLORIDE.—Nausader	19
BACH.—Acorus root—a good bitter tonic .	31
CHIRETTA.—Stems of Swertia chirata—a well-known good tonic	55
CHOBCHINI.—Root of Smilax china—a good alterative	56
GULANCHA.—Stems of Tinospora—a good alterative and tonic like Calumba .	75
MUDAR.—Root of Calotropis gigantea—a good bitter tonic	95
SARSAPARILLA (INDIAN).—Root of Hemidesmus—a good tonic and alterative	118

Anthelmics.

Antiscorbutics.

Antispasmodics.

Antispasmodics—*concld.*

Astringents.

Astringents—*concld.*

Carminative, Aromatic Stimulants, Stomachics.

Carminative, Aromatic Stimulants, Stomachics—*concld.*

Demulcents.

Diuretics.

Emetics.

Expectorants.

Expectorants--*concld.*

Purgatives.

Sedatives and Narcotics.

Sherbets and Cooling Drinks.

Stimulants.

Stimulants—*concld.*

Tonics.

Tonics—*concld.*

Local.

Local—*concld.*

CHAPTER II.

SOURCE, ACTION, AND METHOD OF USE OF THE MOST COMMON AND USEFUL BAZAAR MEDICINES.

AJOWAN—OMUM SEEDS—CARUM.

The seeds of Carum and Ptychotis Ajowan.

A very good digestive, an aromatic, pungent stimulant, digestive and antispasmodic.

Four preparations are available in the bazaar—

(1) The seeds. Known as Ajowan bij.
(2) Ajowan-ki-phul. A crystalline substance.
(3) Ajowan-ki-tel. A distilled oil.
(4) Ajowan-ki-arrack. Omum water.

A substance identical to thymol can be got from the oil.

℞		
	Ajowan seeds	
	Rock salt (*Sendha nimak*)	equal parts— 1 dram
	Asafœtida (*Hing*)	
	Chubelic myrobalans (*Har, chhoti*)	

Dose:—10 grains after food.

For dyspepsia and colic.

℞ Ajowan seeds . 3 lb., in a cloth bag.
Water . . 6 quarts.

Distil in a small still for 4 or 5 hours. This is Omum water.

Dose:—1 ounce.

For spasmodic colic, flatulency, diarrhœa and vomiting of cholera and cholera.

℞		
Ajowan-ki-tel . .	2	minims.
Mucilage . . .	½	dram.
Water	½	ounce.

For flatulent colic.

℞		
Omum water . . .	1	ounce.
Lime water . . .	1	ounce.
Tinct. opii . . .	5	minims.

For diarrhœa.

℞		
Ferri sulph. (*Kasis*) .	1	grain.
Omum water (*Ajowan-ki-arrack*) . . .	1	ounce.
Infus. chiretta . .	1	ounce.

Twice daily. A good tonic.

℞		
Ajowan seeds (powdered)	½	dram.
Cardamom (powdered) .	1	dram.
Black pepper (powdered)	½	dram.
Ginger (powdered) . .	½	dram.

Dose:—1 dram twice daily.

Carminative and for colic.

ALOES—MUSABAR.

The dried and inspissated juice from the leaves of Aloes socotrina or the Indian bazaar varieties—Aloes indica or Aloes litoralis.

The Indian bazaar varieties need to be purified by boiling in water, allowing to stand for twelve hours, then straining, then mixing the liquors, and set aside in an open vessel till evaporated to dryness.

A good purgative; not suitable for pregnancy or piles or children.

Dose:—2 to 5 grains of powdered Aloes.

℞ Aloes (*Musabar*) . . 24 grains.
Sulphate of iron (*Kasis*) . 24 grains.
Cinnamon (*Dalchini*) . 60 grains.
Honey, *q.s.* for making pill mass.

Divide into 24 pills.

Dose:—1 or 2 pills.

For constipation.

℞ Aloes (*Musabar*) . . 20 grains.
Asafœtida (*Hing*) . . 20 grains.
Honey, *q.s. fiat* pill mass.

Divide into 12 pills.

Dose:—1 pill twice daily.

For hysterical fits and flatulency.

℞ Aloes (*Musabar*) . . 18 grains.
Sulphate of iron (*Kasis*) . 30 grains.
Honey, *q.s.* for a pill mass.

Divide into 24 pills.

Dose:—1 pill three times a day and gradually diminish.

For constipation.

℞ Aloes (*Musabar*) . . 2 grains.
Ginger (*Sonth*) . . 2 grains.
Soap, *q.s.* for one pill.

Dose:—1 pill before food for indigestion.

ALUM—PHITKARI.

A valuable medicine, obtainable in all bazaars. Indian alum occurs as transparent crystals, darker than imported alum due to a trace of iron. It is a good astringent. Useful locally for diseases of the skin, eyes, nose, genitals, rectum. Internally for hæmorrhage, diarrhœa, whooping-cough and asthma.

℞	Aluminis (*Phitkari*) .	3	grains.
	Water	1	ounce.

A lotion for sore eyes.

An injection for gleet.

℞	Alum (*Phitkari*) . .	2	drams.
	Decoction galls . .	1	pint.

Local application for piles.

For prolapse of anus.

Injection for vaginitis and leucorrhœa.

℞	Alum (powdered)	equal parts—5 grains.
	Catechu (powdered)	
	Cinnamon (powdered)	

A powder for diarrhœa.

℞	Alum (*Phitkari*) . .	10	grains.
	Tinct. opii . . .	7	drops.
	Water	1	ounce.

For hæmorrhage from stomach and lungs.

℞ Alum.

In crystal.

Apply to scorpion bite.

℞			
℞	Alum (*Phitkari*) . .	2	drams.
	Milk	1	pint.

Boil for 10 minutes and strain for making whey.

Dose:—2 ounces every 3 hours.

For hæmorrhage, albuminuria and diabetes.

℞			
℞	Aluminis (*Phitkari*) .	5	grains.
	Aqua rosæ . . .	½	ounce.

Twice daily for asthma and cough.

℞			
℞	Aluminis (*Phitkari*) .	2	drams.
	Sugar	2	drams.
	Decoction galls . .	1	pint.

Gargle for tonsillitis and spongy gums.

℞			
℞	Aluminis (*Phitkari*) .	20	grains.
	Water	1	ounce.

For sores on penis.

℞			
℞	Aluminis (*Phitkari*) .	1	dram.
	Boracis (*Sohaga*) . .	1	dram.
	Water	10	ounces.

Lotion for weeping eczema.

AMMONIUM CHLORIDE—NAUSADER.

An impure variety can be obtained in most bazaars. It can be purified and made into a pure powder by dissolving in hot water and evaporating to dryness and then bottling.

It has the same therapeutic action as the drug of the British Pharmacopœia.

It is a good expectorant and is useful in pharyngitis, laryngitis and bronchitis. It is also good as an inhalant. It increases the secretion. It is also of use in gastric catarrh and want of action of the liver. It promotes bile. It also relieves the pain of migraine and sciatica.

℞ Ammon. chlor. (*Nausader*) 1 dram.
Heated on a dish.
For an inhalation in laryngitis.

℞ Ammon. chlor. (*Nausader*) 20 grains.
Infus. sarsaparilla . . 1 ounce.
For want of action of liver.
For chronic rheumatism.

℞ Ammon. chlor. (*Nausader*) 15 grains.
Aqua camph. (*Kapur pani*) 1 ounce.
For neuralgia and headache.

℞ Ammon. chlor. (*Nausader*) 10 grains.
Simple syrup . . 1 dram.
Aqua anisi . . . 1 ounce.

For bronchitis.

℞ Ammon. chlor. (*Nausader*) 10 grains.
Syrup of orange . . 2 drams.
Inf. of senna (*Sonnamakki*) 1 ounce.

For congested liver.

℞ Ammon. chlor. (*Nausader*) 1 dram.
Methylated spirit . . 1 ounce.
Water . . . . 6 ounces.

A lotion for putting on swollen testicles.

℞ Ammon. chlor. (*Nausader*) 10 grains.
Ext. glycyrrhizæ liq. . 20 minims.
Aqua ad. . . . 1 ounce.

For bronchitis.

℞ Ammon. chlor. (*Nausader*) 2 drams.
Hot water . . . 1 pint.

A fomentation for glands, joints and boils.

ANISEED—ANISE FRUIT—SONF.

The dried fruit of Pimpinella anisum. A good aromatic stimulant, and carminative, obtainable in all bazaars. A useful addition to all cough mixtures.

℞	Aniseed (*Sonf*) . .	2	drams.
	Water	2	pints.

Distil to 1 pint.

Dose :—1 ounce t.d.s.

An antispasmodic for cough.

℞	Aniseed (*Sonf*) . .	½	dram.
	Myrobalans (*Har*) . .	1	dram.
	Sugar	1	dram.

A laxative powder.

℞	Aniseed (*Sonf*) . .	½	ounce.
	Caraway (*Jira*) . .	½	ounce.
	Parched.		

Dose:—1 teaspoonful after meals, as a digestive.

℞	Honey	1	dram.
	Aniseed water . .	1	ounce.

For cough.

ARUSHA—VASAKA—ADHATODA

The root and the leaves of Adhatoda vasica. A good expectorant and antispasmodic for bronchitis, asthma and whooping-cough.

℞	Fresh juice of Arusha leaves	1	ounce.
	Honey . . .	1	ounce.

Dose:—1 to 2 teaspoonfuls.

For cough.

℞	Arusha leaves (dried) .	1	ounce.
	Boiling water . .	1	pint.

Make infusion.

Add	Ginger (*Sonth*) . .	30	grains.
	Pepper (*Kala mirch*) .	30	grains.
	Sugar	2	drams.

Dose:—1 ounce t.d.s.

For chronic bronchitis and asthma.

℞	Arusha root powder .	4	drams.
	Gilo powder (*see* page 76)	4	drams.
	Water	8	ounces.

Make decoction.

Dose:—1 ounce t.d.s.

For bronchitis.

℞ Arusha leaves (dried).

Make cigarettes for asthma.

Official preparations:

Tinct. Adhatoda or Tinct. Vasaka are also useful.

ASAFŒTIDA—HING.

A gum-resin obtained from root of Ferula fœtida. A good antispasmodic and stimulant used in flatulent distension, hysteria and cholera. It can be obtained in most bazaars. The strongly smelling kind is best.

℞			
℞	Asafœtida (*Hing*) . .	1	grain.
	Pepper (*Mirch*) . .	1	grain.
	Opium (*Afim*) . .	¼	grain.
	Camphor (*Kapur*) . .	1	grain.

A pill in diarrhœa and cholera.

℞			
℞	Asafœtida (*Hing*) . .	20	grains.
	Aloes (*Musabar*) . .	20	grains.
	Honey, *q.s.* to make 12 pills.		

Dose:—1 pill twice daily.

For flatulency and hysteria.

℞			
℞	Asafœtida . . .	30	grains.
	Water or thin gruel .	6	ounces.

An enema in flatulent colic.

℞			
℞	Asafœtida . . .	5	grains.
	Soap, *q.s.* for 1 pill, *t.d.s.*		

For nervousness.

℞ Asafœtida (*Hing*) . .	1	grain.
Maschi (*Kastori*) . . .	3	grains.
Gum (*Gond*) . . .	30	grains.
Cinnamon water . .	1½	ounces.

For hysteria.

℞ Asafœtida . . .	4	drams.
Boiling water . .	1	pint.

Rub down, strain and cool.

Dose:—1 tablespoonful t.d.s.

For hysteria and flatulency.

℞ Cinnamon (*Dalchini*) .	1	dram.
Asafœtida (*Hing*) . .	4	drams.
Water	1	pint.

Rub down, then steam and cool.

Dose:—1 tablespoonful.

For spasmodic colic.

℞ Asafœtida (*Hing*)
Ginger (*Sonth*)
Black pepper (*Kala mirch*)
Long pepper (*Pipul*)
Ajowan seeds (*Ajowan*)
Cummin seeds (*Jira*)
Rock salt (*Sendha nimak*)
} equal parts —2 drams.

Dose:—10 to 20 grains, as a digestive.

℞ Asafœtida
Rock salt
Cardamom
Ginger } equal parts—1 grain.

For flatulency of children.

℞ Asafœtida (*Hing*)
Ajowan (*Ajowan*)
Rock salt (*Sendha nimak*)
Chubelic myrobalans (*Har*) } equal parts —2 drams.

Dose:—10 grains.

For colic pain.

℞	Asafœtida (*Hing*) . .	15 grains.
	Yolk of an egg . .	one.
	Water	3 ounces.

For an enema.

For distension of bowel.

ASOKA BARK.

The bark of Saraca indica. It is a strong astringent. Chiefly used to check uterine hæmorrhage and hæmorrhage of piles.

℞	Asoka bark . . .	4	ounces.
	Milk	4	drams.
	Water	16	ounces.

Boil to a quarter and strain. It must be made fresh every day.

Dose:—1 ounce t.d.s.

A tincture is also made.

The pounded flowers are sometimes used.

ATIS.

The root of Aconite heterophyllum. A valuable tonic after malarial fever, a good febrifuge, good bitter tonic. It is a small tuberous root about 1 inch long, wrinkled, grey in colour. It should be white on breaking across.

℞	Atis radix (powdered) .	30	grains.

Dose:—1 powder three times a day during fever.

℞	Atis powder	5	grains.
	Sugar	10	grains.

Dose:—1 powder t.d.s. as a tonic.

℞	Atis powder (*Atis*) . .	4	drams.
	Ginger (*Sonth*) . .	4	drams.
	Kurchi (*Kurchi*) . .	4	drams.
	Root of Tinospora (*Gulancha*)	4	drams.
	Water	1	pint.

Boil down to a quarter.

Dose:—1 to 2 ounces, as a tonic, t.d.s.

℞	Atis (*Atis*)	equal parts —10 grains.
	Kaladana (*Kaladana*)	
	Black pepper (*Kala mirch*)	
	Ginger (*Sonth*)	

Dose:—5 grains twice daily.

A laxative and tonic.

BABERANG—EMBELIA RIBES

The fruit of Embelia ribes and Embelia robusta. Small globular seeds, obtainable in bazaars. A good anthelmic for tape-worm.

℞	Baberang powder . .	1 dram.
	Sugar	1 dram.

One dose on an empty stomach for tape-worm.

BABUL GOND—GUM BABUL.

Babul-ki-chhal—Indian Gum Arabic.

The bark of Acacia arabica. A mild astringent. Generally used locally, but a decoction also can be made. Contains tannin.

℞ Babul bark (bruised) . 2 ounces.
Water . . . . 1 pint.

Boil for 10 minutes and strain. (Decoction.)

A good application for protruding piles, prolapse of rectum, a gargle for spongy gums, and a lotion for leucorrhœa and gonorrhœa.

℞ Alum (*Phitkari*) . . 1 dram.
Decoction Babul . . 1 pint.

For gargle or for piles.

BACH OR ACORUS ROOT.

The root of Acorus calamus. A thick flat spongy root with aromatic odour and bitter taste. A good bitter tonic and stomachic.

℞	Acorus root (*Bach*), (bruised)	1	ounce.
	Boiling water . . .	10	ounces.

Infuse for 6 hours.

Dose:—1 ounce t.d.s.

A bitter tonic.

℞	Bach root . . .	1	ounce.
	Chiretta stems . .	1	ounce.
	Water	1	pint.

Infuse for 6 hours.

Dose:—1 ounce t.d.s.

A good tonic.

℞	Bach (bruised) (*Acorus root*)	2	ounces.
	Coriander (*Dhania bij*) .	1	dram.
	Kala mirch (*Pepper*) .	½	dram.
	Water	1	pint.

Boil down to 12 ounces and cool.

Dose:—1 ounce t.d.s.

For dysentery ; 2 *teaspoonfuls for a child.*

℞	Bach (powdered) . .	1	ounce.

A dusting powder for fleas, lice and vermin.

BAEL FRUIT—BEL (Hindi).

The fruit of Ægle marmelos, obtainable in most bazaars. The half-ripe fruit is the best. The unripe fruit is astringent. The ripe fruit is lightly aperient. A good remedy for dysentery.

The fresh watery preparations from pulp and Bael sherbet are generally used. It contains little tannin.

"Dietetic Bael" and fluid extract of Bael are good preparations which can be got from the chemist (Bathgate & Co., Calcutta).

℞ Bael fruit (the gummy
 interior) . . . . 2 ounces.
 Water . . . . 4 ounces.

Mix and add sugar.

Dose:—One such three times a day; 2 teaspoonfuls for a child.

For dysentery and scurvy.

BAEL SHERBET.

℞ Pulp of 4 Bael fruits.

Boiling water . . .	1	pint.

Allow to cool and add sugar.

Dose:—2 ounces every 3 hours.

For dysentery and sprue.

℞		
Bael fruit, unripe (powdered)	5	grains.
Pulv. kino co. . .	2	grains.
Sugar	2	grains.

Twice daily for diarrhœa.

℞		
Bael fruit (powdered) .	5	grains.
Butea gum (*Palas-ki-gond*)	5	grains.
Pulv. cinnamon . . .	5	grains.

For diarrhœa.

BETEL LEAF—PAN.

The fresh leaves of Piper betel. Contains an aromatic oil and astringent.

(1) Pan is a mastigatory for chewing. It contains small quantities of—

Lime (*Chuna*).
Catechu (*Katha*).
Betel-nut (*Supari*).
Cardamom (*Ilachi*).
Nutmeg (*Jaiphal*).
Cloves (*Long*).
Camphor (*Kapur*).

Wrapped in betel leaf.

Said to be stimulant, tonic, digestive.

(2) Betel leaves warmed and smeared with oil make a good poultice over the liver and in bronchitis.

BETEL-NUT—ARECA-NUT—SUPARI.

The kernel of the fruit of Areca catechu. It is astringent and carminative. It is one of the constituents of Pan. It is also a vermifuge.

℞	Areca-nut (powdered) .	10	grains.
	Sugar	10	grains.

Dose:—1 powder t.d.s.

To check diarrhœa.

℞	Areca-nut powder (*Supari*)	40	grains.
	Lemon juice . . .	4	drams.

For vermifuge.

℞	Areca-nut powder (*Supari*)	4	drams.
	Milk	4	ounces.

For tape-worm.

℞ Areca-nut powder.

Burn till charred.

A tooth-powder.

℞	Areca-nut powder (*Supari*)	2	drams.
	Catechu (*Katha*) . .	2	drams.
	Cinnamon (*Dalchini*) .	30	grains.

A tooth-powder.

BHINDI—ABELMOSCHUS—EDIBLE HIBISCUS.

The fresh unripe capsules are used. It yields a viscid mucilage on decoction. It is a good demulcent.

℞	Bhindi capsules . . .	3	ounces.
	Water	1	pint.

Boil for 20 minutes.

Dose:—2 to 3 ounces frequently.

For irritable bladder and gonorrhœa.

The inhalation of the steam from above decoction relieves bronchitic cough.

BONDUC-NUT—KATKALIJA.

The seed of Cæsalpinia bonducela. An oval nut, ½ inch long, grey colour. The seeds are used without the shells. A good febrifuge and antiperiodic and tonic.

℞ Bonduc seed (powdered) . 10 grains.
Black pepper . . . 5 grains.

Dose:—1 powder twice daily.

A tonic for intermittent fever and debility.

BHOREE LOTH—THOONIA LOTH.

The leaves of Combretum pilosum, a shrub of Cachar. Anthelmic.

℞	Powdered leaves . .	2 ounces.
	Water	1 pint.

Boil for 20 minutes.

Dose:—2 oz. preceded and followed by a dose of castor oil.

BORAX—SOHAGA.

Can be purchased in most bazaars. A crystal line mass covered with a white powder. A good sedative, Borax is milder and more sedative than Boracic Acid, as it is alkaline.

℞ Boracis (*Sohaga*) . . 1 dram.
Honey . . . . . 1 ounce.

For thrush and sore tongue and ulcers on mouth.

℞ Boracis (*Sohaga*) . . 1 ounce.
Glycerine . . . 5 ounces.

Makes Glycerine of Borax.

For a mouth wash.

℞ Boracis (*Sohaga*) . . 4 drams.
Water . . . . . 8 ounces.

For a gargle, also for sore nipples.

℞ Boracis
Oxide zinc } equal parts.
Starch

A dusting powder.

℞ Glycerine of Borax
Cinnamon water } equal parts.

For painting ulcerated throat.

℞ Boracis . . . . 1 dram.
Simple ointment . . 1 ounce.

For simple ulcers, sore nipples and inflamed piles.

℞ Glycerine Borax . . 4 drams.
Peppermint water . . 6 ounces.

For a mouth wash and gargle.

℞ Boracis . . . . 4 drams.
Camphor water . . 8 ounces.

A lotion for pruritus of genitals, skin irritation and ulcers.

℞ Boracis . . . . 2 drams.
Water . . . . 1 pint.

For an eye lotion.

℞ Boracis . . . . 10 grains.
Cinnamon powder . . 10 grains.

Dose:—1 powder t.d.s.

For uterine inertia and irregular menses.

℞ Boracis
Sulphur
Catechu } equal parts— 1 dram.
Ung. simplex . . . 1 ounce.

For parasitic ulcers.

℞ Boracis (*Sohaga*)
Common salt (*Nimak*) } equal parts— 10 grains.

Dissolve in 8 ounces of water.

Sniff up nose for nasal catarrh.

BUTEA SEEDS—PALAS-KI-BIJ (Hind.).

Seeds of Butea frondosa. A good anthelmic for round-worms. Seeds obtainable in most bazaars.

Seeds are soaked in water and testa removed. Kernel is powdered.

℞		
Kernel of Butea seeds	. 20	grains.
Sugar	. 10	grains.

One such dose t.d.s. for three days, then castor oil.

For round- or tape-worm.

BUTEA GUM—PALAS-KI-GOND (Hind.).

The gum of Butea frondosa—the bazaar kino. A good astringent, like catechu.

℞	Butea gum (powdered) .	15 grains.
	Cinnamon powder . .	5 grains.

For diarrhœa ; in smaller dose for dyspepsia.

CAMPHOR—KAPUR.

A sublimed volatile oil from wood of Cinnamomum camphora. White masses with strong smell, well known in the bazaar.

INTERNALLY a nerve sedative antispasmodic, a cardiac stimulant, carminative, diaphoretic.

EXTERNALLY anodyne.

A valuable bazaar medicine; can be well taken in milk.

℞	Camphor (*Kapur*) . .	1 dram.
	Water	1 pint.

Allow to stand for 2 days—" Camphor water ".

Dose:—A wineglassful.

A diaphoretic vehicle for other drugs.

℞	Camphor (*Kapur*) . .	1 ounce.
	Kurua tel . . .	4 ounces.

A good liniment for lumbago and sciatica, chest and sprains.

℞	Camphor (*Kapur*) . .	3 grains.
	Pil. opii (*Afim*) . .	½ grain.

For chordee, spermatorrhœa, pruritus, chronic rheumatism, internal pains.

℞	Camphor (*Kapur*) . .	3 grains.
	Asafœtida (*Hing*) . .	3 grains.

Dose:—1 pill twice daily.

For asthma, delirium and insomnia.

℞ Camphor (*Kapur*) . . . 1 grain.
Asafœtida (*Hing*) . . 1 grain.
Pil. opii (*Afim*) . . ½ grain.

For diarrhœa and ptomaine poisoning.

℞ Camphor . . . 1 grain.
Oxide zinc
Boracis
Starch
} equal parts—2 drams.

Powder for prickly heat, or sloughing ulcer.

℞ Camphor . . . 1 ounce.

Heated on a plate.

For a vapour bath.

℞ Camphor
Musk
Honey
} equal parts—1 grain in pill.

In late stages of fever and exhaustion.

℞ Camphor (*Kapur*) . . ½ dram.
Ung. boracis (*Sohaga*) . 1 ounce.

A good ointment for pruritus and eczema of genitals.

℞ Camphor (*Kapur*) . . . 1 grain.
Ipecac. powder . . ¼ grain.

For diarrhœa.

CAPSICUM—CHILLIES—LAL MIRCH.

The dried fruit of Capsicum minimum. A powerful rubefacient and counter-irritant. A good stomachic, carminative and stimulant.

℞	Capsici (*Lal mirch*) . .	1	grain.
	Rhei (*Revanchini*) . .	5	grains.
	Ginger (*Sonth*) . .	5	grains.

A good stomachic powder.

℞	Capsici (*Lal mirch*) . .	1	grain.
	Asafœtida (*Hing*) . .	1	grain.
	Camphor (*Kapur*) . .	1	grain.

For severe diarrhœa.

℞	Capsici (*Lal mirch*) . .	1	dram.
	Salt (*Nimak*) . . .	4	drams.
	Boiling water . . .	1	pint.

A good gargle for relaxed throat.

℞	Capsici (*Lal mirch*) . .	1	grain.
	Aloes (*Musabar*) . .	1	grain.
	Honey, *q.s.* for a pill.		

For constipation and dyspepsia.

℞ Pulv. capsici (*Lal mirch*) . 1 grain.
Pil. saponis . . . . 3 grains.

One after each meal.

For dyspepsia.

℞ Capsici . . . . . 4 drams.
Ung. simplex . . . 1 ounce.

A stimulating ointment.

℞ Capsici . . . . . 4 drams.
Emplastrum saponis . 1 ounce.

Counter-irritant.

CARAWAY SEEDS—JIRA (Hind.).

The dried fruit of Carum carui. Can be obtained in most bazaars. It is a stimulant, antispasmodic, carminative, aromatic.

℞ Caraway seeds (*Jira*), powdered
Ginger (*Sonth*)
Rock salt (*Sendha nimak*)
Long pepper (*Pipul*)
Pepper (*Kala mirch*)
} *āā* ½ ounce.

Dose:—30 to 60 grains. ½ to 1 teaspoonful after food.

A very good digestive powder.

℞		
Rhei	16	grains.
Sodæ bicarb. . . .	16	grains.
Aqua carui . . .	2	ounces.

Dose:—1 teaspoonful.

For child's digestive.

℞ Caraway seeds (*Jira*)
Dill (*Soya*)
} *āā* 1 ounce, parched.

Dose:—1 teaspoonful after each meal.

A good digestive.

℞		
Caraway seeds (*Jira*) .	3	drams.
Boiling water . . .	10	ounces.

Strain and cool—"Caraway water".

Dose:—1 ounce.

As a digestive.

CARDAMOM—ILACHI.

The dried ripe fruit of Elettaria cardamomum and Ammon. cardamomum, obtainable in all bazaars. A good carminative and stomachic and flavouring agent.

℞		
	Cardamom seeds (*Ilachi*)	equal parts—2 drams, powdered.
	Ginger (*Sonth*)	
	Cloves (*Long*)	
	Caraway (*Jira*)	

Dose:—½ a teaspoonful.

As a digestive.

℞		
	Cardamom seed	equal parts—4 drams, parched.
	Aniseed	
	Caraway seed	

Dose:—1 teaspoonful after each meal.

For dyspepsia.

CASTOR OIL—ARANDI-KE-TEL.

The expressed oil of Ricinus communis is obtainable in all Indian bazaars. The dark brown oil is acrid in taste. Pale straw colour is the best. It is used for the same diseases and in the same manner as detailed in the British Pharmacopœia. In India it is especially valuable as an emulsion in infantile diarrhœa and irritative diarrhœa of adults and in dysentery.

℞ Castor oil . . . 1 ounce.

A purgative for adults.

One teaspoonful for infants.

℞ Castor oil . . 5 drops.
Mucilage (*gond*) . 5 drops.
Water . . . 1 teaspoonful.

For infantile diarrhœa.

℞ Castor oil . . 1 teaspoonful.
Laudenum . . 5 drops.

For chronic diarrhœa b.d.s. for an adult.

℞ Castor oil . . . 2 drops.

Into eye for sand or grit.

CATECHU—KATHA.

The extract from wood of Acacia catechu. It is obtained by boiling and inspissating the decoctions. It can be bought in most Indian bazaars in brown masses. It is used in Pan. It is an astringent for diarrhœa, ulcers, sore throats and stomatitis.

℞			
℞	Catechu (*Katha*) . .	10	grains.
	Cinnamon powder (*Dalchini*)	10	grains.
	Syrup, *q.s.* to make pill mass.		

Divide into 4 pills.

Dose:—1 pill t.d.s.

For diarrhœa.

℞			
℞	Catechu (*Katha*) . .	3	drams.
	Cinnamon (*Dalchini*) . .	1	dram.
	Boiling water . . .	10	ounces.

Infuse for 2 hours and strain.

Dose:—1 ounce t.d.s.

For diarrhœa.

℞			
℞	Catechu (*Katha*) . .	30	grains.
	Copper sulph. (*Kasis*) .	10	grains.
	Ung. simplex . . .	1	ounce.

An astringent ointment.

℞	Catechu	5	drams.
	Water, hot . . .	1	pint.

A lotion for sore nipples and old ulcers.

℞	Catechu	5	grains.

Put under the tongue.

For sore throat and spongy gums and mercurial stomatitis.

℞	Catechu (*Katha*) . .	1	dram.
	Chalk (*Kharimatti*) . .	1	dram.
	Alum (*Phitkari*) . .	1	dram.
	Ferri sulph. (*Kasis*) . .	30	grains.
	Gall-nut powder (*Maiphul*)	1	dram.

A tooth-powder.

℞	Catechu (*Katha*) . .	2	drams.
	Myrrh (*Bol*) . . .	1	dram.
	Chalk (*Kharimatti*) . .	4	drams.
	Oil of cloves . . .	3	drops.

A good tooth-powder.

CHARCOAL—KOYLAH.

Deodorant and disinfectant, obtainable in all bazaars.

℞	Charcoal (*Koylah*) . .	1	ounce.
	Rice flour . . .	4	ounces.

Add boiling water till consistency of a poultice.
For foul ulcers.

℞	Charcoal (*Koylah*) . .	5	grains.
	Rhei (powdered) . .	5	grains.

Dose:—1 powder after food.
For dyspepsia.

℞	Charcoal (*Koylah*) . .	5	grains.
	Ginger	5	grains.
	Rhubarb . . .	2	grains.

Powder for indigestion.

℞	Charcoal (finely powdered)	equal parts.
	Areca-nut (*Supari*)	
	Chalk (*Kharimatti*)	

A tooth-powder.

℞	Charcoal (*Koylah*) . .	5	grains.
	Bicarbonate of soda .	10	grains.

For dyspepsia.
Dose:—1 powder at each meal.
For heartburn.

CHAULMOOGRA OIL—CHAULMOOGRA TEL.

The oil expressed from the seeds of Gynocardia odorata, obtainable in most bazaars. A remedy for leprosy, lupus, chronic eczema. Used both externally and internally. A fattening tonic in debility.

℞	Chaulmoogra oil . .	2	ounces.
	Nim oil	2	ounces.

Rub into lepric spots.

℞	Chaulmoogra oil . .	5	drops.
	Mucilage . . .	1	dram.
	Syrup	1	dram.
	Water	4	drams.

Dose:—For 1 dose. In leprosy. Twice daily after food. Gradually increase dose.

℞	Chaulmoogra oil . .	5	drops.
	Warm milk . . .	1	ounce.

Dose:—Twice daily after food as a tonic.
For leprosy.

℞	Chaulmoogra seeds (powdered)	5	grains.
	Saponis, *q.s.* for a pill.		

Dose :—1 pill t.d.s.
For leprosy and eczema.

℞ Chaulmoogra oil . . .	5	drops.
Cod-liver oil . . .	30	drops.
Mucilage . . .	1	dram.
Water	1	ounce.

Dose:—1 ounce t.d.s.

For leprosy.

℞ Chaulmoogra oil . .	1	dram.
Ung. simplex . . .	1	ounce.

Ointment for chronic eczemic and lepric spots.

Chaulmoogra oil is also used hypodermically with great benefit for leprosy.

CHIRETTA.

The dried plant of Swertia chirata or Ophelia chirata. It is collected when in flower. It is obtainable in all bazaars. A good, bitter tonic. Useful for indigestion and torpid liver and tonic after fevers.

℞	Chiretta (bruised) . .	1	ounce.
	Boiling water . . .	1	pint.

Infuse for 6 hours and strain.

Dose:—2 ounces t.d.s.

As a tonic.

℞	Chiretta	1	ounce.
	Cloves (powdered) . .	1	dram.
	Cinnamon (powdered) .	1	dram.
	Boiling water . . .	1	pint.

Infuse for 6 hours and strain.

Dose:—2 ounces before food, twice daily.

℞	Chiretta	2	ounces.
	Sherry wine . . .	1	bottle.

Let it stand for 1 week.

Dose:—A wineglassful, once daily before food.

As a tonic.

℞	Ferri sulph. (*Kasis*) . .	4	grains.
	Syrup of orange . .	2	drams.
	Infusion chiretta . .	2	ounces.

A good tonic.

CHOBCHINI—CHINA ROOT.

The root of Smilax china. Imported from China and obtainable in Indian bazaars.

An alterative like Sarsaparilla.

℞ Chobchini	. . .	2 ounces.
Water	. . . .	1 pint.

Boil down to 10 ounces.

Dose:—1 ounce t.d.s.

As a tonic.

CINNAMON—DALCHINI.

The dried inner bark of stocks of Cinnamomum zeylanicum—a large, thick bark, obtainable in most bazaars. The Indian country cinnamon is most inferior.

It is a good stomachic, carminative and tonic. It is also a heart stimulant, and antispasmodic. Useful in flatulency, dyspepsia, diarrhœa, dysentery and fevers.

℞	Cinnamon powder (*Dalchini*)	1	dram.
	Myrobalans (*Har*) . .	4	drams.
	Water	4	ounces.

Boil for 10 minutes.

A good aromatic purge.

℞	Cinnamon (bruised) (*Dalchini*)	1	dram.
	Catechu (*Katha*) . .	3	drams.
	Boiling water . . .	10	ounces.

Macerate for 2 hours and strain.

Dose:—2 teaspoonfuls t.d.s.

For diarrhœa.

℞	Cinnamon powder . .	4	grains.
	Catechu	4	grains.

An astringent powder for diarrhœa.

℞	Ginger (*Sonth*) . .	10	grains.
	Cinnamon (*Dalchini*) .	10	grains.
	Cardamom (*Ilachi*) . .	10	grains.

Dose:—1 powder before food.

For dyspepsia and flatulency.

℞	Cinnamon (*Dalchini*) .	1	dram.
	Cloves (*Long*) . . .	10	grains.
	Ginger (*Sonth*) . .	30	grains.

For one powder.

Boil in 1 seer water for 15 minutes—"Influenza infusion".

Dose:—2 ounces every 3 hours.

For influenza. Very good indeed for influenza.

℞	Cinnamon (*Dalchini*) .	1	dram.
	Aniseed (*Sonf*) . .	½	dram.
	Liquorice (*Mulathi*)		
	Raisins without stone (*Manaka*) . . .	1	dram.
	Sweet almond (*Badam sherif*)	3	drams.
	Bitter almond without rind (*Badam tulkhe*) .	1	dram.
	White sugar (*Misri sufed*) .	1	dram.

Powder all well together and make a pill mass. Divide into 5-grain pills.

Dose:—1 pill several times a day.

For cough.

CLOVES—LONG.

The dried flower buds of Eugenia caryophyllata. They can be obtained in all bazaars. A good stimulant and carminative for indigestion, flatulency and colic.

℞			
℞	Cloves (bruised) . .	3	drams.
	Boiling water . . .	1	pint.

Infuse and strain—"Infusion of Cloves".

Dose:—1 ounce t.d.s.

For flatulency.

℞			
℞	Infus. cloves . . .	4	ounces.
	Infus. chiretta . .	4	ounces.

Dose:—1 ounce b.d.s.

A tonic in flatulency.

℞			
℞	Cloves (bruised) . .	5	drams.
	Sodæ bicarb. . . .	20	grains.
	Hot water . . .	1	wine-glass.

Take before meal.

For indigestion.

℞			
℞	Cloves	30	grains.
	Ginger	30	grains.
	Senna leaves . . .	1	ounce.
	Boiling water . . .	10	ounces.

Allow to stand for 1 hour and strain.

A good aromatic purgative.

℞	Sodæ bicarb. . . .	15	grains.
	Ginger	5	grains.
	Infus. cloves . . .	1	ounce.

Antacid and carminative.

For indigestion.

COPPER SULPHATE—NILA TUTIYA—TUTIA.

A good astringent and emetic. It is obtainable in most bazaars.

℞ Copper sulphate crystal (*Nila tutiya*)

Apply to granular lids and exuberant ulcers.

℞	Copper sulph. (*Tutia*)	2 to 4	grains.
	Alum (*Phitkari*) . .	2	grains.
	Water	1	ounce.

A lotion for conjunctivitis, gleet and leucorrhœa injection.

℞	Copper sulph. (*Tutia*) .	6	grains.
	Opium (*Afim*) . . .	6	grains.
	Honey, *q.s.* for pill mass.		

Divide into 12 pills.

Dose:—1 pill t.d.s.

For chronic diarrhœa.

℞	Cupri sulph. . . .	5	grains.
	Water	1	pint.

An emetic for adults in opium poisoning.

℞ Cupri sulph. . . .	5	grains.
Water	1	ounce.

Dose:—1 teaspoonful.

An emetic for children in diphtheria and bronchitis.

℞ Cupri sulph. . . .	1	dram.
Rose water . . .	6	ounces.

Lotion for prickly heat.

CORIANDER SEEDS—DHANIA.

The seeds of Coriandrum sativum. The seeds are aromatic, carminative, antispasmodic and contain a volatile oil.

℞	Coriander seeds (*Dhania*)	2	drams.
	Water, boiling . .	1	pint.

Infuse for an hour.

Dose:—1 ounce t.d.s.

For flatulency.

℞	Coriander seeds (*Dhania*)	4	drams.
	Sugar	2	drams.
	Milk	1	pint.

Boil for 10 minutes.

Dose:—2 ounces.

For flatulency and piles.

℞	Coriander seeds (*Dhania*)	equal parts, parched.
	Cardamom powder (*Ilachi*)	
	Caraway powder (*Jira*)	

Dose:—1 teaspoonful after food.

As a digestive. A very good remedy.

CREAT OR KIRYET (Hindi), KALMEG (Bengali).

The dried stem and roots of Andrographis paniculata, obtainable in all bazaars. A good, bitter tonic, stomachic, febrifuge, anthelmic and gentle aperient for flatulency and loss of appetite and debility.

℞			
℞	Creat stems (cut up)	4	drams.
	Acorus (*Bach*)	1	dram.
	Dill seeds (*Soyah*)	1	dram.
	Water, boiling	½	pint.

Infuse for 1 hour and strain.

Dose:—1 ounce t.d.s., before food.

For dyspepsia.

℞			
℞	Creat	2	ounces.
	Alcohol	60	per cent.

By percolation to 1 pint to make a tincture.

Dose:—½ to 1 dram.

For influenza.

℞			
℞	Creat	3	ounces.
	Myrrh	4	drams.
	Brandy	1	pint.

Macerate for 7 days, shake, strain, press and filter.

Dose:—1 teaspoonful t.d.s.

For dyspepsia.

CROTON SEEDS—JAMALGOTA.

The seeds of Croton tiglium, obtainable in all bazaars. They should be fresh. A powerful gastro-intestinal irritant. A good local rubefacient. The expressed oil from seeds generally used.

℞	Croton oil (*Jamalgota tel*) .	4	drams.
	Mustard oil (*Rai-ki-tel*) .	6	ounces.

A good liniment for bronchitis and rheumatism.

℞	Croton oil . . .	4	drams.
	Cocoanut oil . . .	4	ounces.

A liniment for chronic rheumatism.

℞	Croton oil . . .	1	drop.
	Sugar	1	dram or a lump.

A powerful purgative for cerebral hæmorrhage or convulsions.

CUBEBS—KABABCHINI.

The dried full-grown unripe fruit Piper cubeba. Small black seeds, obtainable in most bazaars. The size of black pepper.

It is an expectorant and diuretic. It stimulates the secretion of the respiratory and urino-genitary tract. Also a carminative.

℞		
℞	Cubebs (powdered) (*Kababchini*)	30 grains.
	Alum (powdered) (*Phitkari*)	5 grains.

Dose:—1 powder t.d.s.

For gleet and gonorrhœa.

℞		
℞	Cubebs	10 grains.
	Mucilage . . .	30 drops.
	Cinnamon water . .	1 ounce.

Dose:—1 ounce t.d.s.

For bronchitis and laryngitis.

℞		
℞	Cubebs	10 grains.
	Pot. nit. . . .	10 grains.

Dose:—1 powder b.d.s.

For gonorrhœa.

℞		
℞	Cubebs (*Kababchini*) .	1 ounce.
	Sugar	1 ounce.
	Syrup orange . . .	2 drams.
	Water	1 ounce.

Dose:—1 teaspoonful thrice daily.

For gleet.

DATURA.

The dried leaves of Datura alba and fatuosa. It is obtainable in all bazaars. A narcotic, anodyne and antispasmodic. Chiefly used for relief of asthma. Seeds are used by poisoners in sweetmeat or hooka.

℞	Dried datura leaves	. 15	grains.
	Smoked in a pipe.		

For asthma and paroxysmal cough.

The fresh leaves, bruised into pulp with water, can be mixed with a poultice and used for painful joints or lumbago.

℞	Datura leaves . . .	1	ounce
	Boiling water . . .	1	pint.

For use as a hot fomentation.

For dysmenorrhœa, lumbago and pleurodynia.

A tincture and extract can be obtained from chemists and is useful in mania, excitement and tetanus.

DILL—SOYAH.

The dried fruit of Peucedanum graveolens, obtainable in all bazaars. A good aromatic, carminative and stimulant.

℞	Dill seeds (*Soyah*) . . .	3 drams.
	Boiling water . . .	10 ounces.

Infuse till cold and strain.

This is Dill water.

Dose:—1 to 4 teaspoonfuls.

For flatulency.

℞	Dill water . . .	4 ounces.
	Lime water . . .	4 ounces.

Dose:—½ ounce.

For flatulency and abdominal pain.

℞	Dill water . . .	1 ounce.
	Aniseed water . . .	1 ounce.
	Lime water . . .	1 ounce.
	Syrup	½ ounce.

Dose:—1 to 2 teaspoonfuls.

For children's flatulency.

FENNEL—BARI SONF.

The dried ripe fruit of Fœniculam vulgari—a stomachic and carminative.

R	Fennel fruit (*Bari sonf*) (powdered) . . .	20	grains.
	Bael fruit (powdered) .	1	dram.

Dose:—powder t.d.s.

For dysentery.

℞	Fennel fruit (*Bari sonf*)	equal parts, 2 drams.
	Ginger (*Sonth*)	
	Caraway (*Jira*)	

Dose:—½ teaspoonful after food.

A food digestive.

℞	Fennel fruit (*Bari sonf*) .	½	dram.
	Myrobalans . . .	1	dram.

Dose:—For a purgative.

GALLS—MAIPHUL—MAJUFAL.

Excrescences on Quercus infectoria due to deposition of eggs of Cynips gallæ tinctoria, obtainable in all bazaars. Black and blue varieties are best. A powerful astringent.

℞ Galls (bruised) . . . 2 ounces.
Water . . . . 1 pint.

Boil for 10 minutes.

Doles—1 ounce.

For diarrhœa and internal hæmorrhage.

Also useful as an astringent gargle, application for painful piles and prolapse of rectum.

And an injection for prolapse of uterus.

℞ Galls (powdered) (*Maiphul*) 15 grains.
Opium powder (*Afim*) . ½ grain.
Cinnamon powder (*Dalchini*) 5 grains.
Honey, *q.s.* for a pill.

For chronic diarrhœa.

℞ Galls (powdered) (*Maiphul*) 2 drams.
Opium (*Afim*) . . . ½ dram.
Ung. simplex . . . 1 ounce.

Ointment for piles.

℞ Alum (*Phitkari*) . . 1 dram.
Honey or syrup . . 4 drams.
Decoction galls . . . 8 ounces.

Gargle for tonsillitis and sore throat.

GARJAN TEL—WOOD OIL.

An oleo-resin or balsam from Dipterocarpus turbinatus. It is obtainable in most bazaars. A good demulcent, acting on the mucous membrane of the bronchial tubes like copaiba.

℞	Garjan tel . . .	1 dram.
	Malt extract . . .	½ ounce.

For bronchitis, b.d.s.

℞	Garjan tel . . .	1 dram.
	Mucilage	1 dram.
	Lime water . . .	4 drams.
	Water	1 ounce.

For leprosy, b.d.s.
Also a good external application.

℞	Garjan tel . . .	1 dram.
	Mucilage	1 dram.
	Dill water . . .	1 ounce.

For gonorrhœa and gleet, acts like copaiba.

GINGER—SONTH.

The dried root of Zingiber officinale. A strong aromatic stimulant, stomachic and carminative.

℞ Ginger (*Sonth*) (bruised) . 1 ounce.
Boiling water . . . 1 pint.

Infuse for one hour and strain—"Infusion of ginger".

Dose:—1 ounce.

For flatulency and colic.

℞ Ginger . . . . 1 ounce.
Brandy . . . . 8 ounces.

Leave for 10 days.

Dose:—1 teaspoonful in water or added to other medicine as carminative and stimulant.

℞ Sodæ bicarb. . . . 30 grains.
Infus. ginger . . . 2 ounces.

Dose:—2 ounces.

For dyspepsia and vomiting.

℞ Ginger (powdered) . . 1 ounce.
Water, *q.s.* for a plaster.

Apply for headache and face-ache.

℞ Ginger powder . . 1 ounce.

Rub into leg in cramp.

℞ Ginger . . . . 1 grain.
Sodæ bicarb. . . . 3 grains.
Rhubarb . . . 2 grains.

For a child's digestive.

℞ Ginger powder . . 2 grains.
Ferri sulph. . . . 2 grains.
Rhubarb . . . 2 grains.

Dose:—1 powder after food as a tonic t.d.s.

℞ Ginger (*Sonth*) . . 10 grains.
Ajowan (*Ajowan*) . . 1 dram.
Cardamom powder (*Ilachi*) 30 grains.

Dose:—1 powder after food b.d.s.

For indigestion.

℞ Ginger (*Sonth*) . . 2 drams.
Brandy . . . . 4 ounces.
Leave for 7 days.
Add syrup . . . 6 ounces.

Dose :—2 teaspoonfuls for carminative and flavouring agent.

GROUND-NUT OIL—(MONKEY-NUTS) MUNGPHALI TEL.

Made from fruit of Arachis hypogæa, obtainable in all bazaars. The nuts are very nutritive, having starch 37%, oil 11% and albuminous matter 31%. Owing to their richness, they cause biliousness if taken in excess. The ground-nut oil (Arachis oleum) is a very good substitute for olive oil for all liniments and preparations. It is about one-fourth the price and so good for district work. It is a mild aperient.

GULANCHA—TINOSPORA CORDIFOLIA.

The dried stems collected during the hot season, obtainable in most bazaars. A good, bitter tonic, diuretic and alterative and antiperiodic. Good substitute for Calumba.

℞	Gulancha (bruised)	1	ounce.
	Water (cold)	½	pint.

Macerate for 3 hours and strain.

Dose:—1 ounce t.d.s. as a tonic.

For dyspepsia after fevers.

℞	Gulancha (*Gulancha*)	1	dram.
	Chiretta (*Chiretta*)	1	dram.
	Ginger (*Sonth*)	1	dram.
	Water	1	pint.

Boil down to half.

Dose:—1 ounce after fever as a tonic.

℞	Gulancha (*Gulancha*)	1	dram.
	Cloves (*Long*)	1	dram.
	Cinnamon (*Dalchini*)	1	dram.
	Water	1	pint.

Boil down to half.

Dose:—1 ounce t.d.s.

For dyspepsia.

GILA-KA-SAT or SAT-GILO is a white powder sold in the bazaar, obtained by powdering the stem and extracting the starch with water ; said to be a good tonic and bladder sedative.

Dose:—1 dram with milk and sugar.

ISAPHGUL.

The seeds of Plumbago ovata. They yield a demulcent and astringent infusion on soaking in water. A good demulcent, of great use in dysentery, diarrhœa and cystitis.

℞			
℞	Isaphgul seeds . .	2	drams.
	Water (cold) . . .	8	ounces.

Infuse all night.

Dose:—2 teaspoonfuls of the swollen seeds t.d.s.

For dysentery and cystitis.

℞			
℞	Isaphgul seeds (powdered)	1	dram.
	Aniseed (*Sonf*). . .	30	grains.
	Sugar	30	grains.

For one powder.

Dose:—Take 1 powder t.d.s.

For dysentery.

℞			
℞	Isaphgul seeds (powdered)	1	dram.
	Indrajat (*Kurchi seeds*)	5	grains.

Dose:—1 powder.

For dysentery.

℞			
℞	Isaphgul seeds (powdered).	1	dram.
	Pot. nit. . . .	10	grains.
	Cubebs	15	grains.

Dose:—1 powder b.d.s.

For gonorrhœa.

℞	Isaphgul seeds (bruised)	. 2	drams.
	Water . . .	. 1	pint.

Boil for 10 minutes.

Dose:—2 ounces t.d.s.

For cystitis.

"Isaphgul-ka-chilka" is the mucilaginous shells of the seeds and can be bought in the bazaar.

Dose:—1 teaspoonful in 2 ounces of warm water.

JANGLI PIKVAN—VOMITING SWALLOW WORT—ANANTAMUL (Bengali).

The leaves and root of Tylophora asthmatica. A good emetic and expectorant, a substitute or Ipecac. in dysentery. The leaves are more efficacious than root.

℞ Jangli pikvan leaves (powdered)	10	grains.
Pulv. opii . . .	¼	grain.
Mucilage . . .	1	dram.
Aqua	1	ounce.

Dose:—1 ounce t.d.s.

For dysentery and diarrhœa.

℞ Jangli pikvan leaves .	5	grains.
Syrup liquorice . .	30	drops.
Water	4	drams.

Dose:—½ ounce t.d.s.

For bronchitis and whooping-cough.

℞ Jangli pikvan leaves . .	40	grains.

For an emetic.

JATAMANSI—BALCHIR—INDIAN SPIKENARD.

Root of Nardostachys jatamansi. It is obtainable in all bazaars. A good antispasmodic and nervous tonic for hysteria, chorea, convulsions and epilepsy. It is also a good digestive and carminative.

℞	Jatamansi (powdered)	20	grains.
	Camphor (*Kapur*)	3	grains.
	Cinnamon (*Dalchini*)	5	grains.

Dose:—1 powder b.d.s.

For epilepsy and hysteria.

℞	Jatamansi (bruised)	5	ounces.
	Proof spirit	1	pint.

Make a tincture.

Dose:—1 teaspoonful with 10 grains Pot. brom. and 10 drops Tinct. valerian.

For hysteria.

℞	Jatamansi (bruised)	2	drams.
	Boiling water	10	ounces.

Make an infusion.

Dose:—1 ounce t.d.s.

For hysteria, nervousness and convulsions.

KALADANA.

Dried seeds of Ipomœa hedercea, obtainable in all bazaars. A good laxative and purgative.

℞	Kaladana seeds (powdered)	1	ounce.
	Rock salt (*Sendha nimak*)	1	ounce.
	Ginger (*Sonth*) . .	1	dram.

Dose:—1 teaspoonful t.d.s.

As a purgative.

℞	Kaladana (powdered) .	20	grains.
	Black pepper (*Kala mirch*)	5	grains.
	Atis (*Atis*) . . .	15	grains.

Dose:—1 powder.

For feverish attack, twice daily.

KAKMARI—COCCULUS INDICUS SEEDS.

The seeds of Anamirta cocculus. They are very poisonous berries, obtainable in most bazaars. They are the source of Picrotoxin. Internally they strongly irritate the nervous system, causing violent spasm. Should only be used externally and even then not on abraided surfaces.

℞	Kakmari seeds . .	10	grains.
	Ung. simplex . . .	1	ounce.

For pediculi.

℞	Expressed oil of Kakmari seeds	1	dram.
	Cocoanut oil . . .	1	ounce.

For pediculi.

KAMALA.

Powdered capsules of Mallotus philippinensis. A red powder, obtainable in all bazaars. Useful for a remedy for tape-worm and chronic skin disease and ring-worm.

℞ Kamala powder . . 2 drams.
Honey, *q.s.* for one dose.

For tape-worm, repeat in a week.

℞ Kamala (powdered)
Baberang seeds (powdered)
Chhoti Hur
Rock salt (*Sendha nimak*) } equal parts.

Dose:—1 teaspoonful in milk.

For tape-worm.

℞ Kamala . . . . . 4 drams.
Sweet oil . . . . 4 ounces.

Boil. Apply morning and evening.

For ring-worm.

KAKRA SINGHI.

Gall-like excrescences found on Pistacia integerrima and on Rheus succedanea. Much used by Indian physicians. An expectorant and demulcent.

℞	Kakra Singhi (powdered) .	15	grains.
	Ginger (*Sonth*) . . .	5	grains.
	Long pepper (*Pipul*) .	5	grains.

Dose:—1 powder thrice daily.

For cough and influenza.

℞	Kakra Singhi . . .	5	grains.
	Atis	5	grains.
	Pipul	5	grains.
	Honey	1	dram.

A linctus for children.

KOKUM-KI-TEL.

Expressed from seeds of Garcinia purpura. It is a concrete oil, solid when cold. Chiefly composed of tristearin. It is difficult to obtain. It is a very good application to ulcers and cuts. It is applied when warm and fluid, it then solidifies over the ulcer. It is soothing and protective.

KURCHI (BARK) AND INDRAJAB (SEEDS).

The bark and seeds of Wrightea antidysenterica, obtainable in most bazaars. A specific for dysentery.

℞	Kurchi bark (bruised)	. 1	ounce.
	Water (boiling)	. 1	pint.

Infuse for 6 hours and strain.

Dose:—1 ounce t.d.s.

For chronic dysentery.

℞ Indrajab seeds (powdered) 5 grains.

Taken twice daily with Bael decoction.

For dysentery.

Solid and liquid extracts are now made and can be bought from chemists, which are of good value.

LALCHITA—ROSE-COLOURED LEAD WORT—RAKTO-CHITA (Bengali).

The root of Plumbago rosea, common in Indian gardens. A powerful painful vesicant.

℞	Lalchita (fresh bark of root)	4	drams.
	Rice flour	1	ounce.
	Water, *q.s.* to make a paste.		

Spread on cloth, apply to skin for 10 to 20 minutes. Then apply a poultice for 6 hours, to make a blister.

LEMON GRASS OIL—GANDHA-BENA TEL.

Also known as Indian oil of Verbena, though it only resembles Verbena. It is the oil distilled from Andropogon citratis and is obtainable in all bazaars. A good rubefacient liniment. Internally a stimulant and carminative. Useful in vomiting and cholera.

℞	Gandha-bena tel . . .	5	drops.
	Mucilage . . .	30	drops.
	Aqua cinnamon . .	4	drams.

For flatulent colic and vomiting.

℞ Gandha-bena tel . . . 5 drops.

On sugar.

For vomiting.

℞	Gandha-bena tel . .	4	ounces.
	Sweet oil . . .	4	ounces.

A liniment. Apply locally.

For lumbago and rheumatism.

LIME—SLAKED LIME—CHUNA.

Freshly prepared by interaction of water and calcium oxide (unslaked lime). Sedative and astringent, antacid.

℞ Slaked lime . . . . 1 ounce.
Water . . . . . 4 pints.

Shake well in a stoppered bottle and allow to stand for 12 hours.

Use as lime water.

To prevent curdling of milk.

For diluting milk.

For acidity and heartburn, pyrosis.

For vomiting.

℞ Slaked lime . . . . 2 ounces.
White sugar . . . . 2 ounces.
Water . . . . . 1 pint.

Shake and allow to stand.

Dose:—20 drops.

For antacid in childhood, with milk or before food.

℞ Lime water } equal parts—
Aqua } 4 ounces.

For pruritus valve or vaginal injection and cracked nipples.

℞	Lime water Glycerine Water	equal parts.

For itching of the skin.

R	Lime water Olive oil	equal parts.

For burns, scalds, cracked nipples and eczema.

℞	Calomel (*Hydrarg. subchlor.*)	30	grains.
	Lime water . . .	½	pint.

Black wash for foul sores and gargle.

℞	Lime water . . .	2	ounces.
	Sweet oil . . .	2	ounces.
	Carbolic acid . . .	10	drops.

For burns, scalds and small-pox pustules.

LIME JUICE—NIMBU.

Fresh juice of Citrus acida. Limes can be got at the right season in the bazaars. A good anti-scorbutic and refrigerant drink.

℞ Fresh lime juice . . 1 ounce.
Sugar . . . . 2 drams.
Water . . . . 8 ounces.

Dose:—One such drink twice daily.

For scurvy.

℞ Fresh lime juice . . 4 ounces.
Water . . . . 4 ounces.

A gargle for spongy gums. Also antidote to castor-oil and croton-oil poisoning.

℞ One lime cut in pieces . 1 lime.
Sugar . . . . 4 drams.
Barley water . . . 1 pint.

A cooling drink.

℞ Fresh lime juice.

Apply locally for mosquito bites.

LINSEED—ULSI.

The seeds of Linum usitatissimum. The seeds yield a rich oil on pressure. On soaking in water they give a viscid mucilaginous jelly-like mass. A good demulcent.

LINSEED TEA. As a demulcent in colds, cough, dysentery and cystitis. Take 1 ounce linseed, clean it by picking out all other seeds. Boil in 1 pint of water for 5 to 10 minutes and strain. Add sugar.

Dose:—½ pint twice daily.

For dysentery, cough and cystitis.

LINSEED POULTICE. Take a basin and warm it. Add boiling water 6 to 8 ounces, sprinkle linseed on the water and stir; add till the mixture is like thick porridge or suji. Press and mash the mixture against the side of the basin while hot. Pour the mixture on to a piece of cloth, spread with spatula making it ¼ inch thick. Smear surface with oil.

Apply to the chest while hot.

℞	Lime water	. . .	2 ounces.
	Linseed oil	. . .	2 ounces.

For application to burns.

LIQUORICE—MULATHI.

The root of Glycyrrhizæ glabra. It is not indigenous to India, but is obtainable in all bazaars. The root of Abrus precatorious is often sold in its stead. It is demulcent and expectorant.

℞		
℞	Liquorice root . . .	2 ounces.
	Bhindi capsules . .	1 ounce.
	Water	1 pint.

Boil for half an hour and strain. Add sugar 8 ounces, boil down to a syrup.

Dose:—1 to 4 teaspoonfuls.

For troublesome cough.

℞		
℞	Liquorice (*Mulathi*)	equal parts—1 dram for a pill mass.
	Camphor (*Kapur*)	
	Asafœtida (*Hing*)	
	Gum babul (*Gond babul*)	

Dose:—5 grains for a pill.

For influenza and cough.

MANGOSTIN.

The fruit of Garcinia mangostana. Largely imported into Indian bazaars. A good astringent and antidysenteric. The rind and the whole fruit is used medicinally. It contains tannin.

℞	Mangostin rind . . .	2	ounces.
	Water	1	pint.

Boil for half an hour and strain. Make a decoction. Add syrup 4 drams.

Dose:—1 ounce t.d.s.

For dysentery.

℞	Mangostin fruit (dried and powdered) . . .	10	grains.
	Cinnamon powder (*Dalchini*)	5	grains.
	Cardamom (*Ilachi*) . .	10	grains.

Dose:—1 powder t.d.s.

For dysentery.

℞	Mangostin powder . .	10	grains.
	Cubebs (*Kababchini*) .	10	grains.
	Alum (*Phitkari*) . .	10	grains.
	Gum acacia (*Gond*) . .	10	grains.

A sedative powder for gonorrhœa.

MUDAR (Hindi); AKANDA (Bengali).

The dried root-bark of Calotropis procera and Calotropis gigantea, free from outer corky layers. It should be gathered in April and May from plants grown in sandy soil and dried without the sun, before peeling off the bark.

A good tonic, alterative, expectorant. In big doses an emetic and gastro-intestinal irritant, a substitute for Ipecacuanha.

℞ Mudar (powdered) . . 4 grains.
Ginger (*Sonth*) . . . 4 grains.

Dose :—Powder t.d.s.

As a tonic and expectorant.

Also said to be good for leprosy.

℞ Mudar powder . . . 20 grains.

A good emetic or given for dysentery with a previous dose of Tinct. opii and on empty stomach and mustard plaster to epigastrium.

MUSK—KASTURI.

The pod of secretion from preputial follicles of musk-deer, obtainable in bazaars of Northern India.

A stimulant in low fevers and debility and chronic coughs. Combined with other stimulants and antispasmodics.

℞ Nutmeg (*Jaiphal*)
Mace (*Jaipatri*)
Long pepper (*Pipul*)
Black pepper (*Kala mirch*)
Musk (*Kasturi*)
} equal parts—in pill.

Dose:—2 grains.

℞ Musk (*Kasturi*)
Cardamom (*Ilachi*)
Clove (*Long*)
Date (*Khurma*)
} equal parts—5 grains.
Honey . . . . 1 ounce.

Dose:—One teaspoonful.

For a stimulant and a remedy for hoarseness.

℞ Musk (*Kasturi*) . . 1 grain.
Camphor (*Kapur*) . . 3 grains.

In a pill for depression.

MUSTARD—RAI.

The prepared commercial mustard can be bought in most bazaars; also the expressed oil from seeds. A good condiment. A powerful irritant and rubefacient. In large doses an emetic.

℞	Mustard (*Rai*) (prepared)	1	ounce.
	Water	8	ounces.

Dose:—This draught for an emetic.

Useful in narcotic poisoning.

℞	Mustard (*Rai*) . . .	½	ounce.
	Boiling water . . .	1	gallon.

For foot bath.

℞	Mustard (prepared) . .	½	ounce.
	Flour or Linseed meal .	8	ounces.

Add boiling water and stir to form a poultice (see *Linseed poultice*). *A most efficient application in pleurisy, pneumonia, hepatitis and rheumatism.*

℞	Mustard (prepared) . .	10	ounces.
	Hot water in bath . .	10	gallons (40 seers).

Place the feet or whole body in bath; a warm mustard bath is most stimulating. Good for headache, common colds, convulsions.

℞ Oil of mustard (*Rai*) . . ½ dram.
Camphor (*Kapur*) . . 1 dram.
Castor oil . . . . 2 drams.
Alcohol . . . . 2 ounces.

A good stimulating liniment.

℞ Oil of mustard . . 4 drops.
Methylated spirits . . 1 ounce.

Paint on back of ear in discharge from ear.

MYROBALANS (BELERICA)—BAHERA.

The dried fruit pulp without stones of Terminalia belerica, obtainable in all bazaars. Astringent and laxative, used also for loosening coughs and hoarseness.

℞		
	Bahera . . .	equal parts —½ ounce.
	Sendha nimak . .	
	Pipul . . .	
	Kala mirch . .	

Honey, *q.s.* for a linctus.

Dose:—1 dram.

For cough.

℞		
	Bahera . . .	equal parts —2 drams.
	Anwala . . .	
	Har	
	Pipul	
	Black salt . . .	
	Sugar	

Dose:—½ to 1 dram.

As a digestive.

MYROBALANS (EMBELIC)—ANWALA-AWLA.

The fresh and dried fruit of Phyllanthus emblica. The fresh fruit is diuretic and laxative and a good cooling sherbet may be made from it. The dried fruit is astringent and useful in diarrhœa and dysentery.

℞	Anwala (juice of fresh fruit) . .	3	drams.
	Sugar	3	drams.
	Water	10	ounces.

For a sherbet, diuretic and laxative.

℞	Anwala powder . .	4	drams.
	Har	4	drams.
	Rhubarb powder . .	1	dram.
	Water	1	pint.

Boil for 10 minutes.

Dose:—2 ounces.

For indigestion and laxative.

MYROBALANS (CHUBELIC)—HAR OR CHHOTI HAR.

Obtainable in all bazaars. The dried immature fruit of Terminalia chebula. Two varieties are met with, Chhoti Har and Bari Har. The former is used for medicinal purposes. The latter for tanning. Chhoti Har is a good laxative, both astringent and aperient. A good tonic and alterative. Makes a good astringent lotion and ointment.

℞		
	Har (powdered) . .	equal parts —½ ounce.
	Long pepper (*Pipul*) .	
	Rock salt (*Sendha nimak*)	

Dose:—30 grains after each meal.

For diarrhœa and a carminative.

℞			
	Myrobalan fruit (*Chhoti har*)	6	drams.
	Cinnamon powder (*Dalchini*)	1	dram.
	Cloves powder (*Long*) .	1	dram.
	Water	8	ounces.

Boil for 10 minutes and strain for one dose.

A good purgative.

℞			
	Har (powdered) . .	5	drams.
	Rhei radix (powdered) .	1	dram.
	Water	4	ounces.

Boil for 10 minutes.

A good purgative.

℞	Har (powdered) Ginger (*Sonth*) Aniseed (*Sonf*) Rock salt (*Sendha nimak*)	equal parts —1 dram.

Dose:—10 grains b.d.s.

A digestive and liver alterative, before food.

℞ Har (powdered) . . 2 drams.
Catechu (*Katha*) . . 2 drams.
Sweet oil, *q.s.* to make a paste.

A good astringent application.

℞ Har (powdered) . . 1 dram.
Fennel (*Bari sonf*) . . 1 dram.
Sugar . . . . 1 dram.

Laxative powder, once or twice daily.

MYRRH—BOL.

The gum resin from Balsamo-dendron myrrha, obtainable in bazaars. A mild disinfectant and alterative to mucous membranes, a mild expectorant and uterine stimulant—stomachic, soluble in alcohol.

℞			
℞	Myrrh (*Bol*) . . .	1	dram.
	Honey	1	dram.
	Spt. vin. rectif. . .	1	dram.
	Infus. rosa . . .	6	ounces.

For stomatitis and mouth wash.

℞			
℞	Myrrh (*Bol*) . . .	1	dram.
	Boracis (*Sohaga*) . .	1	dram.
	Syrup	2	drams.
	Water	2	drams.
	Spt. vin. rectif. . .	2	ounces.

Application for thrush.

℞			
℞	Pulv. myrrh . . .	1	grain.
	Ferri. sulph. . . .	1	grain.

In pill, twice daily, as a tonic after food

℞			
℞	Pulv. myrrh . . .	3	grains.
	Pulv. rhei . . .	3	grains.
	Kaladana . . .	5	grains.

As a stomachic.

NIM BARK—NIM.

The dried bark of Melia azad dirachtæ. Though almost every part of the tree is used by Indian physicians medicinally, the bark is practically the only portion of any use. It is a good bitter tonic, astringent, antiperiodic.

℞	Nim bark powder (*Nim*)	½	dram.
	Cinnamon powder (*Dalchini*)	5	grains.

A tonic powder, b.d.s.

℞	Nim bark (bruised) . .	2	ounces.
	Cloves (*Long*) . . .	10	grains.
	Boiling water . . .	1½	pints.

Boil for 15 minutes.

Dose:—2 ounces.

As a tonic.

For loss of appetite and tonic.

℞	Bruised nim leaves . .	1	ounce.
	Rice flour . . .	1	ounce.

Tepid water to make a poultice.

For indolent ulcer and eczema.

Official preparations—

(1) Infusion azad dirachtæ indica ½ ounce.

(2) Tincture azad dirachtæ indica ½ to 1 dram.

NUTMEG—JAIPHUL.

The imported variety is the dried seeds of Myristica fragrans and is obtainable in all bazaars. The country nutmeg is the dried fruit of Myristica malaberica and is not so good. It is an aromatic and carminative.

℞	Jaiphul (powdered) . .	5	grains.
	Caraway (*Jira*) . .	10	grains.
	Ginger (*Sonth*) . .	5	grains.

A carminative before meals.

The oil of nutmeg, which is used in perfumery, when mixed with sweet oil, makes a good liniment for chronic rheumatism.

OPIUM (Afim).

Opium is obtainable in all Indian bazaars. It has the same therapeutic action as the drug of the British Pharmacopœia. The most valuable drug for the relief of pain. Dose ½ to 2 grains.

Poppyheads (the capsules of Papaver somniferum) are used extensively as a sedative fomentation and poultice. The poppyheads are bruised and boiled in water. A flannel is dipped into the hot fluid, wrung out and applied locally.

℞ Opium powder . . ½ grain.
Cinnamon powder . . 5 grains.

For diarrhœa and pain.

℞ Galls (*Maiphul*) . . 2 drams.
Opium (*Afim*) . . . ½ dram.
Ung. simplex . . . 1 ounce.

For piles.

℞ Powdered ginger (*Sonth*) . 1 grain.
Powdered opium (*Afim*) . ½ grain.
Powdered camphor (*Kapur*) 1 grain.

For diarrhœa, flatulency and pain.

PAPAIYA TREE.

The milk juice of the fruit of Carica papaya. A strong digestive.

℞	Milky juice of unripe fruit	1	dram.
	Sugar	1	dram.

Divide into 3 doses.

Dose:—One, three times a day.

For enlargement of spleen.

℞ Slices of unripe fruit.

Rub on ring-worm once daily. Said to cure.

℞ Fresh juice of unripe fruit when dried, forms a powder. Dry in the sun; makes PAPAIN.

Dose:—10 grains.

For dyspepsia.

℞	Papain	10	grains.
	Rhubarb radix (*Revanchini*)	5	grains.
	Cinnamon (*Dalchini*) .	5	grains.

As a digestive powder before meals.

℞	Fresh juice of unripe fruit	½	ounce.
	Honey	½	ounce.
	Boiling water . . .	2	ounces.

A draught for round-worm, followed by castor oil.

PEPPER (BLACK)—KALA MIRCH.

The dried unripe fruit of Piper nigrum. It is obtainable in all bazaars. A good stimulant, stomachic and carminative. Locally a good counter-irritant.

℞		
℞	Black pepper (*Kala mirch*)	2 grains.
	Asafœtida (*Hing*) . .	1 grain.
	Opium (*Afim*) . . .	¼ grain.

For diarrhœa.

℞		
℞	Pepper (*Kala mirch*)	equal parts—2 drams.
	Ginger (*Sonth*)	
	Long pepper (*Pipul*)	
	Caraway (*Jira*)	
	Rock salt (*Sendha nimak*)	

Dose:—½ to 1 teaspoonful.

As a digestive after food.

℞		
℞	Kala mirch	2 drams.
	Caraway powder (*Jira*) .	4 drams.
	Honey	4 ounces.

Rub well together.

Dose:—¼ to 1 teaspoonful.

As a digestive.

℞ Kala mirch . . . 2 drams.
Boiling water . . . 1 pint.

As a good gargle when cold.

℞ Black pepper (*Kala mirch*) ½ dram.
Caraway (*Jira*) . . 1 dram.
Honey or sugar . . 3 ounces.

Make into a paste.

Dose:—1 teaspoonful.

For piles.

Or mixed with equal parts.

Confection of senna.

PIPUL—PIPULI—PIPULI MULA
LONG PEPPER.

The fruit, root and stems of Piper longum. Pipuli mula is applied to the roots and joints of stems—pipul to the catkins. A good stimulant, carminative and alterative, also an expectorant.

℞ Long pepper (*Pipul*)
Ginger (*Sonth*)
Black pepper (*Kala mirch*)
Cinnamon (*Dalchini*)
Caraway (*Jira*)
} equal parts —2 drams.

Dose:—¼ to 1 dram.

A good expectorant powder.

℞		
	Pipul	10 grains.
	Anwala	10 grains.
	Har	10 grains.
	Sendha nimak . .	10 grains.

Dose:—1 powder after food.

A good digestive powder.

An infusion made of 10 peppers with honey makes a good expectorant.

PITHORI—TURBAND—WHITE TURPETH ROOT.

The root and root-bark of Ipomœa turpethum. The black turpeth is not used. A strong purgative well known in the bazaars.

℞	Pithori (*Turband*) . .	30	grains.
	Ginger	10	grains.
	Cream of tartar . .	10	grains.

A strong purgative.

℞	Pithori (*Turband*) . .	40	grains.
	Rock salt (*Sendha nimak*) .	10	grains.
	Ginger (*Sonth*) . .	10	grains.
	Pepper (*Kala mirch*) .	5	grains.
	Water, *q.s.* for a pulp.		

A purgative.

PLANTAIN—BANANAS—KELAH.

The fruit of Musa sapientum. Valuable in the treatment of sprue, diarrhœa and scurvy. It is not well digested by children.

℞	One plantain fruit mashed.		
	Milk	4	ounces.

Taken slowly with a teaspoon, one three times a day.

For dysentery and sprue.

℞	Plantain fruit . . .	2	drams.
	Tamarind pulp . .	4	drams.
	Salt	½	dram.

Mash and mix well.

Take twice daily.

For dysentery and diarrhœa.

POMEGRANATE—ANAR.

"Anar-ki-chhal", or the root-bark and rind of fruit of Punica granatum, is obtainable in all bazaars. It is a valuable astringent, antidysenteric and anthelmic.

"Anar-ka-pani" is a popular cooling beverage made from juice of fresh fruit.

℞			
℞	Rind of Anar fruit (dried)	2	ounces.
	Cloves (bruised) . .	2	drams.
	Water	1	pint.

Boil for 15 minutes and strain.

Dose:—1 ounce t.d.s.

For dysentery and diarrhœa.

℞			
℞	Root-bark of pomegranate (sliced) . . .	2	ounces.
	Water	2	pints.

Boil down to 1 pint.

Dose:—2 ounces fasting. Repeat every half an hour for 4 doses.

For tape-worm.

℞			
℞	Rind of Anar fruit . .	1	ounce.
	Rind of fruit of mangostin	1	ounce.
	Kurchi bark . . .	1	ounce.
	Water	1	pint.

A decoction for dysentery.

Dose:—1 ounce t.d.s.

POTAS. NIT.—SALTPETRE—SHORA (Hindi)—SORA (Bengali).

Impure Pot. nit. is obtainable in most bazaars. It needs to be purified by boiling in water, straining and allowing to recrystallize. A good diuretic and diaphoretic. It has the same therapeutic action and is used for the same purpose as the drug in the English Pharmacopœia. It can easily be combined with many Indian drugs.

℞ Nitre (*Shora*) . . . 10 grains.
Decoction bhindi . . 2 ounces.

For gonorrhœa.

℞ Nitre (*Shora*) . . . 10 grains.
Infus. Moringa root . . 1 ounce.

For dropsy.

℞ Nitre (*Shora*) . . 2 teaspoonfuls.
Barley water . . 1 pint.

For fever.
For a diuretic.

Dose :—One or two tablespoonfuls 3 or 4 times a day.

RASAUT—BARBERRY ROOT—DAR HALDI (Bengali).

An extract, decoction and tincture can be made from the dried bark and root. It is a bitter tonic alterative, astringent and stomachic. In large doses it is aperient.

℞	Rasaut root (chopped) .	6	ounces.
	Water	2	pints.

Boil down to 1 pint.

Dose:—2 ounces every 4 hours.

A diaphoretic and bitter tonic.

Bazaar "Rasaut" is a watery extract of the root. It can be purified by dissolving in alcohol and evaporating to a pillular consistency.

Dose:—30 to 60 grains.

℞	Rasaut	5	grains.
	Kernel of nim seed . .	2	grains.
	Raisin (*Manaka*) . .	10	grains.

To form 3 pills. To be taken at bed time.

For piles.

RING-WORM SHRUB—DADMURDAN.

A good cure for ring-worm and parasitic skin diseases.

℞ Bruised fresh leaves
Ung. boracis or simplex } equal parts.

Rubbed into the skin for ring-worm.

℞ Bruised fresh leaves.
Lemon juice, *q.s.* for a paste.

Rubbed into the skin for ring-worm.

SANDAL-WOOD OIL—CHANDAN TEL.

The oil distilled from wood of Santalum album. It can be got in many bazaars. Only a good oil should be used. It is a stimulant and disinfectant of the genito-urinary tract, also expectorant.

℞ Sandal-wood oil . .	5	drops.
Mucilage . . .	30	drops.
Water	1	ounce.

Dose:—1 ounce t.d.s.

For gonorrhœa and cystitis.

SARSAPARILLA (Indian)—SALSA (Hindi) —ANANTAMUL (Bengali).

The dried root of Hemidesmus indicus. A good alterative tonic and diaphoretic.

℞	Hindi salsa root (bruised) .	1 ounce.
	Boiling water . . .	10 ounces.

Infuse for 1 hour and strain, milk and sugar may be added.

Dose:—1 to 2 ounces.

For debility and indigestion.

SENDHA NIMAK—ROCK SALT.

Obtainable in all bazaars. A dull brownish white crystal—an impure variety of common salt, with a little sulphur and bitumen. It has a distinct laxative action and is a help to digestion.

℞	Sendha nimak . . .	10 grains.
	Kaladana . . .	1 dram.
	Ginger (*Sonth*) . . .	10 grains.

A laxative powder.

℞	Sendha nimak . .	equal parts —2 drams.
	Har . . .	
	Anwala (*Myrobalans*)	
	Pipul . . .	

Dose:—10 grains twice, as a digestive.

Black salt or Kala nimak or "Bit Nun" is prepared by Indian Chemists and Hakeems from Sendha nimak and Anwala.

SODIUM CHLORIDE—COMMON SALT—NIMAK.

Can be obtained in all bazaars. A valuable drug which is not used frequently enough in district dispensary work. It is a good emetic, a good gargle, a good dressing for wounds, a help to digestion, good for rheumatic baths, good for rectal subcutaneous and intravenous injection. A good nasal douche in influenza.

℞	Common salt . . .	1	dram.
	Water (warm) . . .	1	pint.

A good gargle for sore throat.

A good nasal douche for influenza.

Good for rectal or subcutaneous injection.

℞	Sodium chlor. . . .	2	drams.
	Pot. chlor. . . .	6	grains.
	Calcium chlor. . . .	4	grains.
	Water (sterile) . . .	1	pint.

Rogers' mixture for intravenous cholera injection.

℞	Common salt . . .	2	drams.
	Hot water . . .	1	pint.

For vaginal douche.

℞	Common salt . . .	30	grains.
	Warm water . . .	6	ounces.

Inject into back passage for worms (thread).

SHAJNA—MORINGA—HORSE-RADISH TREE.

The fresh root of Moringa pterygosperma. The root is stimulant, digestive, diuretic. Useful as a tonic in recovery from fever. The oil of the seeds is known as Ben oil and is used by perfumers.

℞	Moringa root (powdered) .	1	ounce.
	Boiling water . . .	1	pint.

Infuse for 2 hours and strain. This is "Infusion of moringa".

Dose:—2 ounces t.d.s.

A diuretic in dropsy. Also a good gargle in relaxed throat.

℞	Pot. nit. (*Shora*) . .	10	grains.
	Infus. moringa . .	2	ounces.

A good diuretic for calculi, dropsy and gout.

℞		
	Moringa root (powdered)	equal parts —2 drams.
	Long pepper (*Pipul*)	
	Black pepper (*Kala mirch*)	
	Rock salt (*Sendha nimak*)	
	Caraway (*Jira*)	

Dose:—1 dram b.d.s.

For fever.

℞	Decoction moringa root .	6 ounces.
	Pipul . . .	equal parts—3 drams.
	Kala mirch . .	
	Rock salt . .	

Dose:—1 ounce b.d.s.

For enlarged spleen.

℞	Moringa oil . . .	2 ounces.
	Ground-nut oil . .	2 ounces.

For rheumatic joints.

SENNA—SONNAMAKKI.

Leaves of Cassia lanceolata and Cassia angustifolia. Cultivated in Southern India and obtainable in bazaars. A good laxative.

℞	Senna leaves (powdered) .	4	drams.
	Ginger (bruised) (*Sonth*) .	1	dram.
	Cloves (powdered) (*Long*) .	1	dram.
	Water (boiling) . .	1	pint.

Macerate for 2 hours and strain.

Dose:—1 ounce with milk.

For chronic constipation

℞	Infus. senna . . .	4	drams.
	Infus. chiretta . .	1	ounce.

A tonic and a laxative.

Senna pods are also a valuable laxative. Ten pods are left soaking in cold water all night and the supernatant fluid drunk next morning.

Official preparations—

(1) Confect. senna.

(2) Syrup senna.

(3) Tinct. senna.

℞	Senna leaves (powdered)	10	drams.
	Coriander seed (*Dhania*)	4	drams.
	Tamarind pulp	10	drams.
	Cassia pulp	10	drams.
	Prunes	10	drams.
	Sugar	40	drams.
	Water	100	drams (1½ ounces).

A safe and gentle laxative.

Dose :—1 to 2 teaspoonfuls.

SOMRAJ—VERONICA SEEDS—PURPLE FLEABANE.

The dried seeds of Veronica anthelmintica, obtainable in every bazaar. A good anthelmic.

℞	Somraj seed (bruised)	. 1	dram.
	Honey	. 2	drams.

Repeat again in 2 hours. Follow by castor oil.

SUFED DAMAR—PINEY RESIN.

Resin from the trunk of Vateria indica. A large evergreen tree in Southern India.

A fine resin, not unlike amber, which is met with in the bazaars in irregular masses. Used medicinally and also like copal for making varnishes. A good substitute for ordinary resin and a dressing for ulcers.

℞	Sufed damar . . .	5	ounces.
	Kokum	8	ounces.
	Wax	2	ounces.

Melt by gentle heat and stir; spread on lint.

Good resinous dressing for ulcer.

SULPHUR—GUNDAK (Hindi).

Bazaar sulphur is not fit for internal use, as it is not pure enough. It is suitable for external use. It is a parasiticide.

℞	Sulphur (*Gundak*) . .	1 dram.
	Til oil or olive oil or simple ointment . . .	1 ounce.

Rub in every evening.
For scabies.

℞	Sulphur (*Gundak*) . .	1 ounce.
	Nim oil (*Nim tel*) . .	8 ounces.

A liniment for chronic rheumatism.

℞	Sulphur (*Gundak*) . .	equal parts —1 dram.
	Boracis (*Sohaga*) . .	
	Catechu (*Katha*) . .	
	Ung. simplex . . .	1 ounce.

For parasitic or other ulcers.

Sulphur (*Gundak*) . .	4
Mustard (*Rai*) . .	4
Pot. nit. (*Shora*) . .	1
Rhubarb . . .	1
Honey or sugar . .	64

Rub into a paste.

Dose:—1 teaspoonful for rheumatism.

SULPHATE OF IRON—KASIS—HIRI KASIS.

Obtainable in most bazaars. The green crystals are the best. A good hæmatinic and tonic.

℞	Ferri sulph. (*Kasis*)	. 30	grains.
	Aloes (*Musabar*) .	. 18	grains.
	Honey *q.s.*		

Divide into 24 pills.

Dose:—1 pill t.d.s.

Laxative tonic pill.

℞	Ferri sulph. (*Kasis*)	. 10	grains.
	Spirit of wine .	. 1	ounce.

Apply to skin for erysipelas.

℞	Ferri sulph. (*Kasis*)	. 4	grains.
	Infus. chiretta .	. 3	ounces.

Dose:—1 ounce t.d.s. after food.

For anæmia and debility.

℞	Ferri sulph. (*Kasis*) .	. 24	grains.
	Cinnamon powder (*Dalchini*)	30	grains.
	Black pepper (*Kala mirch*) .	30	grains.
	Honey *q.s.*		

Divide into 12 pills.

Dose:—1 pill b.d.s.

As a tonic.

℞ Ferri sulph. . . . . 6 grains.
Water . . . . 2 ounces.

An enema in bleeding piles and prolapse of anus.

TALMAKHAN—ASTERACANTHA.

A small annual—Hygrophila spinosa—with bright purple flowers growing near water.

The dried herb, seeds, and roots are used. They make a demulcent, diuretic, and cooling bitter tonic.

℞	Talmakhan . . .	1	ounce.
	Boiling water . . .	1	pint.

Boil for 10 minutes and strain.

Dose:—2 ounces t.d.s.

For dropsy.

℞	Dried leaves of Talmakhan	2	ounces.
	Vinegar	1	bottle.

Macerate for 3 days, press and strain.

Dose:—½ to 1 ounce t.d.s.

A demulcent diuretic.

℞	Talmakhan root . .	1	ounce.
	Water	1	pint.

Boil for 10 minutes.

Dose:—1 ounce t.d.s.

As a diuretic.

TAMARIND—IMLI.

The fruit of Tamarindus indica.

A refrigerant, laxative and antiscorbutic.

℞	Tamarind fruit (*Imli*) .	1	ounce.
	Dates (*Khurma*) . .	1	ounce.
	Milk	1	quart.

Boil and strain.

A good laxative.

℞	Tamarind fruit pulp .	1	ounce.
	Water	1	pint.

Macerate and strain.

Add	Cloves (powdered) . .	1	dram.
	Cardamom (powdered) .	1	dram.
	Camphor (powdered) .	3	grains.

For loss of appetite.

For a cooling sherbet.

For scurvy.

TURMERIC—HALDI (Hindi).

The dried root stock of Curcuma longa.

Obtainable in all bazaars. An aromatic carminative. Useful in flatulence and dyspepsia. Used largely as a colouring agent.

℞	Turmeric . . .	10 grains.
	Pipul	10 grains.
	Kala mirch . . .	5 grains.
	Ginger	10 grains.
	Cardamom . . .	10 grains.

A simple digestive.

℞	Turmeric (*Haldi*) . .	½ ounce.
	Hemp (*Ganja* leaves) . .	½ ounce.
	Linseed oil, *q.s.* to make a paste.	

For relief in piles.

It is used extensively by Indian physicians for sore eyes, eczema and skin diseases, but its chief value is probably its colour.

TIL OIL—SESAMUM OIL.

The expressed oil of the seeds of Sesamum indicum.

Obtainable in all bazaars. Good substitute for olive oil, for liniments, ointments and plasters.

℞ Til oil . . . . } equal parts.
Lime water . . . . }

For burns and scalds.

TURPENTINE OIL—GANDHE BARAJE-KI-TEL.

The bazaar oil of turpentine is not pure enough for internal use, but is a valuable application externally for rheumatism and as an ointment and for enemata.

℞ Camphor	. . .	½ ounce.
Oil of turpentine	. .	8 ounces.
Soft soap	. . .	1 ounce.

Stir and rub up till well mixed for a liniment.

For rheumatism, sciatica and rubbing on the chest in bronchitis.

℞ Oil of turpentine	. .	1 ounce.
Barley water	. . .	1 pint.

An enema in flatulency, colic spasm and convulsions.

℞ Oil of turpentine	. .	1 ounce.
White damar	. . .	1 dram.
Simple ointment	. .	1 ounce.

For parasites, lice, etc., and indolent ulcers.

℞ Oil of turpentine	. .	2 drams.

Sprinkled on hot flannel.

For stupe in colic, tympanites, cholera and dysentery.

VINEGAR—SIRKA.

Can be bought in most bazaars. It is useful as a cooling agent.

℞ Vinegar . . . 1 ounce.
Water . . . . 4 ounces.

For sponging the body in fevers.

℞ Vinegar . . . } equal parts—
Methylated spirit . } 1 ounce.
Water . . . }

For application to bruises, headache, scorpion-bites, wasp-bites and pruritus.

CHAPTER III.

OVER TWO HUNDRED USEFUL PRESCRIPTIONS OF BAZAAR MEDICINES.

A Bazaar Medical Pharmacopœia.

Abortion.—

℞ Asoka bark . . . 4 ounces.
Milk . . . . 4 ounces.
Water . . . . 1 pint.

Boil down to one-fourth and strain.

One dose t.d.s.

Abortion (inevitable or incomplete).—

℞ Borax (*Sohaga*) . . . 30 grains.
Cinnamon powder (*Dalchini*) 10 grains.

In conjee or arrowroot every 2 hours for three times.

Acidity.—

℞ Slaked lime (*Chuna*) . ½ ounce.
Water . . . . 2 pints.

Shake well and allow to deposit for 12 hours. Mix with equal parts of milk.

Amenorrhœa Pill.—

℞ Asafœtida (*Hing*) . . 1 grain.
Aloes (*Musabar*) . . 1 grain.

One pill twice daily.

Anæmia Pill (1).—

℞ Sulphate of iron (*Kasis*) . 20 grains.
Black pepper (*Kala mirch*) 20 grains.
Honey, *q.s.* for pill mass.

Divide into 10 pills.

Dose:—1 pill twice daily.

Anæmia Pill (2).—

℞ Aloes (*Musabar*) . . 12 grains.
Ferri sulph. (*Kasis*) . . 12 grains.
Cardamom (*Ilachi*) . . 30 grains.
Honey, *q.s.* for pill mass.

Divide into 12 pills.

Dose:—2 pills twice daily.

Antispasmodics (*see* **Carminatives and Digestives).**

Aphthæ (Thrush).—

℞ Borax (*Sohaga*) . . 1 dram.
Honey . . . . . 1 ounce.

Apply with cotton-wool to the mouth.

Asthma.—

℞	Alum	5	grains.
	Rose water	½	ounce.

For asthma b.d.s.

Asthma.—

℞	Camphor (*Kapur*) . .	4	grains.
	Asafœtida (*Hing*) . .	4	grains.

Dose:—1 pill every 3 hours.

Asthma.—

℞	Arusha leaves (dried) .	2	ounces.

Make into cigarettes.

Good substitute for stramonium.

Bed Sores.—

℞	Boracis (*Sohaga*) . .	2	drams.
	Oxide zinc . . .	2	drams.
	Starch	2	drams.

A dusting powder.

Bed Sores.—

℞	Boracis (*Sohaga*) . . .	1	dram.
	Simple ointment . .	1	ounce.

Bed Sores.—

℞	Piney resin (*Sufed damar*)	4	ounces.
	Wax (*Mom*) . . .	2	ounces.
	Lard	8	ounces.

Heat gently and stir while cooling.

Blister.—

℞	Root-bark (*Lalchita*) (fresh)	2	drams.
	Flour of wheat or rice water		sufficient for a paste.

Apply on a cloth to skin for 20 minutes.

Bronchitis.—

℞	Ginger (*Sonth*) . .	5	grains.
	Black pepper (*Kala mirch*)	5	grains.
	Sugar	10	grains.
	Infusion arusha (*Adhatoda*)	1	ounce.

Dose:—1 ounce t.d.s.

Bronchitis (Chronic).—

℞	Jangli Pikvan (*Anantamul*)	5	grains.
	Syrup of country liquorice	1	dram.
	Water	1	ounce.

Dose:—1 ounce t.d.s.

Bronchitis.

℞	Ammon. chlor. (*Nausader*)	10	grains.
	Simple syrup . . .	1	dram.
	Aniseed water . .	1	ounce.

Bronchitis (Chronic) Pill.—

℞	Liquorice root (*Mulathi*) .	1	grain.
	Black pepper (*Kala mirch*)	1	grain.
	Gum babul . . .	1	grain.
	Common salt (*Nimak*) .	1	grain.

Dose:—1 pill t.d.s.

Bronchitis (Chronic).—

℞	Ammon. chlor. (*Nausader*)	1	dram.
	Country liquorice syrup .	2	ounces.
	Water	4	ounces.

Dose:—1 ounce t.d.s.

Bronchitis (Chronic Cough).—

℞	Kakra Singhi . . .	5	grains.
	Triphala (*see* Index) . .	5	grains.

B.d.s.

Bronchitis (Chronic) Cough Pills.—

℞	Liquorice (*Mulathi*) .	equal parts —1 dram.
	Ginger (*Sonth*) . .	
	Ammon. chlor. (*Nausader*)	
	Long pepper (*Pipul*) .	
	Sugar . . .	
	Gum, *q.s.* . .	

Dose:—10-grain pill b.d.s.

Bronchitis (Chronic) "Country Cough Pills".—

℞		
	Kakra Singhi (powdered)	equal parts —1 dram.
	Piplamul (powdered) .	
	Rock salt (powdered) .	
	Gum acacia (*Gond*) .	

Make a pill mass with water.

Dose:—5 grains t.d.s.

Bronchitis Cough Powders.—

℞		
	Kakra Singhi . .	equal parts —1 dram.
	Pipul . .	
	Atis	

Dose:—30 grains t.d.s.

Bronchitis (Chronic) "King of Oudh's Cough Pills".—

℞		
	Cinnamon (*Dalchini*) .	60 grains.
	Aniseed (*Sonf*) . .	60 grains.
	Liquorice (*Mulathi*) . .	60 grains.
	Raisins, without stones (*Manaka*) . . .	180 grains.
	Sweet almonds (*Badam shereef*) . . .	60 grains.
	Bitter almonds without rind (*Badam tulkhe*) .	60 grains.
	White sugar . . .	60 grains.

Powder all drugs well and make into a pill mass.

Dose:—5 grains t.d.s.

Burns.—

℞	Til oil	2	ounces.
	Lime water . . .	2	ounces.

Apply locally.

Camphor Water.—

℞	Camphor (*Kapur*) . .	1	dram.
	Water	1	pint.

Dose:—1 ounce.

Good carminative.

Carminative Powder.—

℞	Chubelic myrobalans (*Har*)	10	grains.
	Embelic myrobalans (*Anwala*) . . .	10	grains.
	Long pepper (*Pipul*) .	10	grains.
	Rock salt (*Sendha nimak*) .	10	grains.

Dose:—1 powder twice daily.

Carminative Powder.—

℞	Ginger (*Sonth*) . .	3	grains.
	Black pepper (*Kala mirch*)	3	grains.
	Fennel fruit (*Bari sonf*) .	5	grains.
	Black salt (*Kala nimak*) .	10	grains.

Dose:—1 powder after food.

Cholera Pill (Incipient).—

℞	Ginger (*Sonth*) . .	3	grains.
	Red pepper (*Lal mirch*) .	1	grain.
	Asafœtida (*Hing*) . .	1	grain.
	Opium (*Afim*) . .	½	grain.
	Camphor (*Kapur*) . .	1	grain.

For one pill—a very good pill.

Chordee.—

℞	Camphor (*Kapur*) . .	4	grains.
	Opium (*Afim*) . .	½	grain.

At bed time occasionally.

Chorea.—

℞	Indian Spikenard (*Jatamansi*)	2	drams.
	Water . . .	1	pint.

Macerate for an hour and strain.

Dose:—2 ounces b.d.s.

Colic.—

℞	Ajowan-ki-tel . . .	2	drops.
	Mucilage . . .	30	drops.
	Water	½	ounce.

Dose:—½ ounce b.d.s.

Colic (Spasmodic).—

℞	Dalchini (*Cinnamon*) .	1	dram.
	Asafœtida (*Hing*) . .	4	drams.
	Water	1	pint.

Rub down, then steam and cool.

Dose:—1 tablespoonful thrice daily.

Colic.—

℞	Ajowan seeds (powdered) .	1	dram
	Cardamom (*Ilachi*) . .	1	dram.
	Black pepper (*Kala mirch*)	30	grains.
	Ginger (*Sonth*) . .	30	grains.

Dose:—1 dram twice daily.

Colic.—

℞	Laudanum	7	drops.
	Omum water (*Ajowan-ki-arak*)	1	ounce.

Colic Pill.—

℞	Asafœtida (*Hing*) . .	2	grains.
	Black pepper (*Kala mirch*)	2	grains.
	Ginger (*Sonth*) . .	2	grains.
	Mucilage acacia (*Gond*), *q.s.* for a pill.		

Twice daily.

Conjunctivitis.—

℞	Alum (*Phitkari*) . .	5	grains.
	Water	1	ounce.

Drops for the eyes twice daily.

Conjunctivitis (Sore Eyes).—

℞	Alum (*Phitkari*) . .	12	grains.
	Zinc. sulphate . .	6	grains.
	Infus. poppyhead . .	6	ounces.

Cracked Nipples.—

℞	Lime water . .	equal parts
	Olive oil . .	—2 ounces.

Contusions (Cooling Lotion).—

℞	Ammon. chlor. (*Nausader*)	2	drams.
	Methylated spirit . .	1	ounce.
	Water	10	ounces.

Convulsions during Labour.—

℞	Borax (*Sohaga*) . .	10	grains.
	Cinnamon (*Dalchini*) (powdered) . . .	10	grains.

Three times a day.

Cooling Drink (Imli Sherbet).—

℞	Tamarind pulp (*Imli*)	1	ounce.
	Sugar	1	ounce.
	Water	1	pint.

Cough.—

℞	Honey	1	dram.
	Aniseed water	1	ounce.

For one dose.

Cough.—

℞	Arusha juice (*Adhatoda*)	1	dram.
	Honey	1	dram.

Linctus for cough.

Dose:—1 teaspoonful.

Cough Pills (*see* **Bronchitis**).

Cystitis.—

℞	Isaphgul seeds	2	drams.
	Water	1	pint.

Boil for 10 minutes and strain.

Dose:—2 ounces t.d.s.

Debility.—

℞	Chiretta (bruised)	2	ounces.
	Sherry wine	1	bottle.

Dose:—½ to 1 wine glass daily.

Debility after Fever.—

℞	Kiryet stem (bruised) .	½	ounce.
	Acorus root (*Bach*) . .	1	dram.
	Dill seeds (*Soyah*) . .	1	dram.
	Boiling water . . .	½	pint.

Infuse for an hour and strain.

Dose:—1 ounce t.d.s.

Delirium and Exhaustion in Fever.—

℞	Camphor (*Kapur*) . .	3	grains.
	Musk (*Kasturi*) . .	3	grains.
	Honey *q.s.*		

Place on the tongue.

Delirium and Exhaustion Pill (Stimulant).

℞	Musk (*Kasturi*) . .	equal parts—5 grains.
	Nutmeg (*Jaiphal*) . .	
	Mace (*Jaipatri*) . .	
	Long pepper (*Pipul*) . .	
	Black pepper (*Kala mirch*)	

Make pill mass.

Dose:—5 grains for 1 pill.

Delirium and Sleeplessness.—

℞	Camphor (*Kapur*) . .	3	grains.
	Asafœtida (*Hing*) . .	3	grains.

Dose:—1 pill at bed time.

Diaphoretic and Antiperiodic.—

℞			
℞	Barberry root (*Rasaut*) .	4	ounces.
	Water	2	pints.

Diaphoretic Powder.—

℞			
℞	Ajowan (*Carum*) . .	8	grains.
	Bark of *Mudar* . .	1	grain.
	Pot. nit. (*Shora*) . .	8	grains.
	Sodæ bicarb. . . .	16	grains.

Dose:—4 grains for a child; 10 grains for an adult.

Diarrhœa.—

℞			
℞	Galls (*Maiphal*) (bruised) .	1	ounce.
	Hot water . . .	1	pint.

Boil for 10 minutes.

Dose :—1 ounce t.d.s.

Diarrhœa.—

℞ Chubelic myrobalans (*Har, chhoti*) . . } equal parts—
Long pepper (*Pipul*) . } ½ ounce.
Rock salt (*Sendha nimak*) }

Dose:—½ teaspoonful after each meal.

Diarrhœa.—

℞	Chalk	2 drams.
	Gum acacia (*Gond*) . .	2 drams.
	Infus. cinnamon . .	8 ounces.

Dose:—1 ounce t.d.s.

Diarrhœa.—

℞	Alum (*Phitkari*) . .	5 grains.
	Catechu (*Katha*) . .	10 grains.
	Cinnamon (*Dalchini*) .	10 grains.

Dose:—1 powder b.d.s.

Diarrhœa and Dysentery.—

℞	Pomegranate rind of fruit (bruised) . . .	2 ounces.
	Cloves (*Long*) . . .	2 drams.
	Water	1 pint.

Boil for 15 minutes and strain.

Dose:—1 ounce t.d.s.

Diarrhœa (Astringent).—

℞	Catechu (*Katha*) .	5—10 grains.
	Cinnamon (*Dalchini*)	5—10 grains.

Dose:—1 powder t.d.s.

Diarrhœa (Astringent).—

℞	Butea gum (*Polas gond*) .	15	grains.
	Cinnamon powder (*Dalchini*) . . .	5	grains.

Dose:—1 powder twice daily.

Diarrhœa.—

℞	Opium powder (*Afim*) .	½	grain.
	Cinnamon powder . .	5	grains.

Dose:—1 powder.

Diarrhœa.—

℞	Camphor (*Kapur*) . .	1	grain.
	Ipecac. powder . .	¼	grain.

Make 8 such. 1 for diarrhœa.

Diarrhœa (Chronic).—

℞	Alum (*Phitkari*) . .	10	grains.
	Laudanum . . .	5	drops.
	Infus. acorus . . .	2	ounces.

Twice daily.

Diarrhœa (Chronic).—

℞	Gall powder (*Maiphal*) .	15	grains.
	Cinnamon (*Dalchini*) .	10	grains.
	Opium (*Afim*) . . .	½	grain.

Dose:—1 powder twice daily.

Diarrhoea (Chronic, of Phthisis).—

℞	Copper sulphate (*Tutiya*)	5 grains.
	Opium (*Afim*) . . .	5 grains.
	Honey, *q.s.* for 10 pills.	

Divide into 10 pills.

Dose:—1 pill b.d.s.

Diarrhoea (of Adults).—

℞	Lime water . . .	1 ounce.
	Laudanum . . .	5 drops.
	Omum water (*Ajowan-ki-arak*)	1 ounce.

Diarrhoea (of Children).—

℞	Copper sulph. (*Tutiya*) .	2 grains.
	Omum water (*Ajowan-ki-arak*)	2 ounces.

Dose:—1 teaspoonful t.d.s.

Diarrhoea or Hæmorrhage (Astringent).—

℞	Catechu (*Katha*) (bruised) .	3 drams.
	Cinnamon (*Dalchini*) .	1 dram.
	Boiling water . . .	8 ounces.

Macerate for 2 hours and strain.

Dose:—2 teaspoonfuls t.d.s.

Diarrhœa Powder.—

℞	Alum (*Phitkari*) . .	4	grains.
	Catechu (*Katha*) . .	5	grains.
	Bael	20	grains.

Dose:—1 powder twice daily.

Digestive Powder.—

℞	Turmeric (*Haldi*) . .	10	grains.
	Long pepper (*Pipul*) .	10	grains.
	Ginger (*Sonth*) . .	5	grains.
	Cardamom (*Ilachi*) . .	10	grains.
	Pepper (*Kala mirch*) . .	5	grains.

Dose:—1 powder b.d.s.

Digestive Powder.—

℞	Chubelic myrobalans (*Har*) .	equal parts of each.
	Embelic myrobalans (*Anwala*)	
	Carum (*Ajowan*) . .	
	Aniseed (*Sonf*) . . .	
	Ginger (*Sonth*) . . .	
	Lahori salt (*Sendha nimak*)	
	Caraway (*Jira*) . . .	
	Common salt (*Nimak*) .	

Dose:—1 to 2 teaspoonfuls after food.

Digestive Powder.—

℞		
	Ginger (*Sonth*) . .	equal parts —2 drams.
	Black pepper (*Kala mirch*)	
	Piper longum (*Pipul*) .	
	Caraway (*Jira*) . .	
	Black salt (*Sendha nimak*)	

Dose:—½ teaspoonful after food b.d.s.

A very good powder indeed.

Digestive Powder.—

℞		
	Ajowan seeds . .	equal parts —1 dram.
	Rock salt (*Sendha nimak*) .	
	Asafœtida (*Hing*) . .	
	Myrobalans (*Har*) . .	

Dose:—1 grain t.d.s.

Digestive Powder.—

℞			
	Ginger (*Sonth*) . .	3	grains.
	Black pepper (*Kala mirch*) .	3	grains.
	Asafœtida (*Hing*) . .	1	grain.
	Black salt (*Sendha nimak*) .	5	grains.

Dose:—1 powder after food.

Digestive Powder.—

℞	Chubelic myrobalans (*Har*)	equal parts —2 drams.
	Ginger (*Sonth*) . .	
	Aniseed (*Sonf*) . .	
	Kurchi	
	Long pepper (*Pipul*) .	
	Rock salt (*Sendha nimak*)	
	Ammon. chlor. . .	

Dose:—1 to 2 teaspoonfuls.

Digestive Powder.—

Triphala	Chhoti Har . .	equal parts —1 dram.
	Bahera . . .	
	Anwala . . .	
	Sugar . . .	
	Pipul . . .	
	Black salt . .	

Dose:—30 grains.

Digestive Powder.—

℞	Sodæ bicarb. . .	equal parts —½ ounce.
	Rhubarb (*Revanchini*) .	
	Ginger (*Sonth*) . .	

Dose:—10 to 30 grains before food.

Digestive Powder.—

℞ Aniseed (*Sonf*) . .	} equal parts	
Caraway (*Jira*) . . .	} —parched.	

Dose:—1 teaspoonful after each meal.

Dropsy.—

℞ Nitre (*Shora*) . . .	10	grains.
Infus. moringa root (*Shajna*)	1	ounce.

Dose:—1 ounce t.d.s.

Dropsy.—

℞ Fresh moringa root . .	1	ounce.
Mustard	1	ounce.
Boiling water . . .	1	pint.

Infuse for 2 hours.

Dose:—1 ounce t.d.s.

Dropsy.—

℞ Barleria root (*Asteracantha*)	1	ounce.
Water	1	pint.

Boil for 10 minutes and strain.

Drink during the day.

Dusting Powder.—

℞ Boracic acid (*Sohaga*) .	2	drams.
Oxide zinc . . .	2	drams.
Starch	4	drams.

Dysentery.—

℞ Mudar root (collected in Spring) . . . 5 grains.
Isaphgul . . . 30 grains.
Sugar . . . . 30 grains.

Dose:—1 powder twice daily.

Dysentery.—

℞ Acorus root (*Bach*) (bruised) 2 ounces.
Coriander seed (*Dhania*) . 1 dram.
Black pepper (*Kala mirch*) 20 grains.
Water . . . . 1 pint.

Boil for quarter of an hour.

Dose:—1 ounce t.d.s.

Dysentery.—

℞ Anantamul leaves (dried) . 10 grains.
Pulv. opii . . . ½ grain.

Dose:—1 powder t.d.s.

Dysentery.—

℞ Castor oil . . . 1 ounce.
Gum acacia . . . 3 drams.
Sugar . . . . 3 drams.
Water, Caraway . . 4 ounces.

Add 1 ounce of the water to the gum. Then add oil gradually and stir. Then add water to 4 ounces.

For adults 15 *drops to* 1 *dram.*

Dysentery.—

℞	Jangli Pikvan (*Anantamul*)	10	grains.
	Tinct. opii . . .	5	minims.
	Mucilage acacia . .	½	dram.
	Water	1	ounce.

Dose:—1 ounce b.d.s.

Dysentery (Acute) Powder.—

℞	Isaphgul (finely powdered)	equal parts.
	Aniseed (finely powdered)	
	Bael (finely powdered) .	

Dose:—½ to 1 teaspoonful twice daily.

Dysentery (Chronic).—

℞	Plantain fruit pulp . .	1	ounce.
	Tamarind pulp . .	4	drams.
	Salt	30	grains.

Mashed up.

Twice daily.

Dysentery (Chronic).—

℞	Kurchi bark . . .	1	ounce.
	Hot water . . .	1	pint.

Infuse for 6 hours and strain.

Dose:—1 ounce t.d.s.

Dysentery (Chronic).—

℞ Alum (*Phitkari*) . . 1 dram.
Mucilage of starch . . 2 ounces.

For an enema. Give slowly.

Dysentery (Chronic) Pills.—

℞ Opium (*Afim*) . . . ¼ grain.
Copper sulph. (*Tutiya*) . ¼ grain.
Camphor (*Kapur*) . . ½ grain.
Mucilage (*Gond*), *q.s.* for 1 pill.

Twice daily.

Dysentery Powder.—

℞ Bael fruit (powdered) . 1 dram.
Fennel fruit (*Bari sonf*) . ½ dram.

Dose:—1 powder twice daily.

Dysentery Powder.—

℞ Bael (powdered) . . 1 dram.
Liquorice (*Mulathi*) . . 10 grains.
Cinnamon (*Dalchini*) . . 5 grains.

Dose:—1 powder twice daily.

Dysentery Powder.—

℞ Isaphgul (powdered) . . 20 grains.
Kurchi seeds (powdered) . 5 grains.

Dose:—1 powder twice daily.

Dysentery Powder.—

℞	
Aniseed powder (*Sonf*)	equal parts —20 grains.
Isaphgul powder .	
Sugar . . .	

Dose:—1 powder twice daily.

Dyspepsia Pill.—

℞	
Capsicum (*Lal mirch*) (powdered) . . .	1 grain.
Soap pill . .	3 grains.

One after each meal.

Dyspepsia.—

℞	
Ajowan seeds (*Carum*) (powdered) . .	equal parts —2 drams.
Rock salt (*Sendha nimak*)	
Asafœtida (*Hing*) .	
Myrobalans (*Har, chhoti*)	

Dose:—10 to 20 grains t.d.s.

Dyspepsia Powder.—

℞	
Ginger (*Sonth*) . .	equal parts —2 drams.
Aniseed (*Sonf*) . .	
Myrobalans (*Har, chhoti*)	
Black salt (*Kala nimak*)	
Salt (*Nimak*) . .	

Dose:—10 to 30 grains after food.

Eczema Lotion.—

℞	Alum (*Phitkari*) . .	1	dram.
	Boracis (*Sohaga*) . .	1	dram.
	Water	8	ounces.

Apply on cloth to the skin.

For Eyes (Sore Lids).—

℞	Borax (*Sohaga*) . .	1	dram.
	Water	½	pint.

Eczema.—

℞	Lime water . .	equal parts.
	Olive oil . . .	

Eczema Powder.—

℞	Sulphur . . .	equal parts —1 ounce.
	Boracis . . .	
	Kamala . . .	
	Sodæ bicarb. . .	

For dusting the part.

Emetic.—

℞	Copper sulphate (*Tutiya*) .	4	grains.
	Water	4	drams.

Dose:—1 teaspoonful every 10 minutes for 4 doses.

11

Emetic.—

℞	Anantamul leaves, dried (Tylophora) . . .	30	grains.
	Sugar	10	grains.

Erysipelas.—

℞	Ferri sulph. (*Kasis*) .	20	grains.
	Spirit of wine . .	2	ounces.

Paint the area.

Expectorant.—

℞	Anantamul leaves (dried) .	5	grains.
	Syrup	1	dram.

One dose t.d.s.

Enema.—

℞	Asafœtida (*Hing*) . .	15	grains.
	Yolk of egg . . .	One.	
	Water	3	ounces.

For flatulent distension.

Eye (Grit in).—

℞	Castor oil . . .	2	drops.

Put under lid.

Eye Lotion.—

℞	Borax	2	drams.
	Water	1	pint.

For bathing sore eyes.

Fever Powder.—

℞	Atis powder	15	grains.
	Bonduc-nut (*Katkalija*) .	15	grains.
	Black pepper (*Kala mirch*)	10	grains.
	Kaladana powder . . .	10	grains.

Dose:—1 powder twice daily.

Fever Powder (Diaphoretic and Laxative).—

℞	Kaladana . .	equal parts —2 drams.
	Atis . . .	
	Black pepper . .	

Dose:—20 grains b.d.s.

Fever Mixture.—

℞	Nitre (*Shora*) . .	2 teaspoonfuls.
	Barley water . .	1 pint (½ seer).

One or two tablespoonfuls three times a day.

Flatulency.—

℞	Aloes (*Musabar*) . .	20	grains.
	Asafœtida (*Hing*) . .	20	grains.
	Honey, *q.s.* for a pill mass.		

Divide into 12 pills.

Dose:—1 pill b.d.s.

Flatulency.—

℞ Oil of turpentine . .	1	ounce.
Barley water . . .	1	pint.

As an enema.

Flatulency (of Children).—

℞ Dill seeds (*Soyah*) (bruised)	3	drams.
Hot water . . .	½	pint.

Infuse till cold and strain.

Dose:—2 or 3 teaspoonfuls.

Flatulency (of Children).—

℞ Caraway seeds (crushed and put in bag) . . .	2	drams.
Boiling water . . .	1	pint.

Boil down to a half.

Dose:—1 to 2 teaspoonfuls.

Flatulency and Colic.

℞ Cinnamon powder (*Dalchini*) . .	equal parts —1 dram.
Ginger (*Sonth*) . .	
Cardamom (*Ilachi*) .	

Dose:—½ teaspoonful b.d.s.

Flatulent Colic.—

℞	Ginger (*Sonth*) (bruised)	. 1	ounce.
	Water	. 1	pint.

Boil for half an hour and strain.

Dose:—1 ounce t.d.s.

Flatulent Colic and Constipation.—

℞	Asafœtida (*Hing*) . .	. 30	grains.
	Water or gruel . .	. 8	ounces.

As an enema.

Foot Bath.—

℞	Mustard (*Rai*) . . .	. ½	ounce.
	Boiling water . .	. 1	gallon.

For a hot foot bath.

Gargle (Astringent).—

℞	Alum (*Phitkari*) . .	. 2	drams.
	Decoction Babul . .	. 1	pint.

Gargles (*see* **Pharyngitis**).

Gonorrhœa.—

℞	Nitre (*Shora*) . . .	. 10	grains.
	Decoction of fresh Abelmoschus (*Bhindi*) . .	. 2	ounces.

Dose:—1 ounce t.d.s.

Gleet.—

℞	Cubebs (*Kababchini*) .	1	ounce.
	Sugar	1	ounce.
	Syrup of orange . . .	2	drams.
	Water	1	ounce.

Gonorrhœa Injection.—

℞	Alum (*Phitkari*) . .	24	grains.
	Water	6	ounces.

For irrigation once daily.

Gonorrhœa Injection.—

℞	Boracis (*Sohaga*) . .	20	grains.
	Water	6	ounces.

Gonorrhœa Powder.—

℞	Cubebs (*Kababchini*) .	30	grains.
	Alum (*Phitkari*) . .	5	grains.

Dose:—1 powder t.d.s.

Gonorrhœa Powder.—

℞	Pulv. cubebs (*Kababchini*)	10	grains.
	Pot. nit. (*Shora*) . .	5	grains.
	Alum (*Phitkari*) . .	5	grains.
	Gum acacia (*Babul gond*) .	10	grains.

Dose:—1 powder twice daily.

Gonorrhœa Powder.—

℞ Cubebs (*Kababchini*) .	20	grains.
Pot. nit. (*Shora*) . .	10	grains.
Sodæ bicarb. . . .	10	grains.

Dose:—1 powder three times a day.

Gonorrhœa with Cystitis.—

℞ Capsules of bhindi (cut up)	3	ounces.
Water	1½	pints.

Boil and strain and add sugar.

A demulcent drink.

Hæmorrhage from Nose.—

℞ Alum (*Phitkari*) . .	2	drams.
Water	6	ounces.

For syringing nose.

Hæmorrhage from Stomach or Lungs.—

℞ Alum	10	grains.
Tinct. opii . . .	5	drops.
Water	1	ounce.

Headache.—

℞ Camphor (*Kapur*) . .	½	ounce.
Vinegar (*Sirka*) . .	8	ounces.
Water . . .	8	ounces.

Apply locally.

Headache (Sick or Bilious).—

℞	Ammon. chlor. (*Nausader*)	10	grains.
	Camphor water . .	1	ounce.

Dose:—1 ounce b.d.s.

Hepatitis and Dropsy.—

℞	Ammon. chlor. (*Nausader*)	20	grains.
	Infus. moringa (*Shajna*)	1	ounce.

Dose:—1 ounce t.d.s.

Hysteria.—

℞	Camphor (*Kapur*) . .	4	grains.
	Asafœtida (*Hing*) . .	4	grains.

Dose:—1 pill b.d.s.

Hysteria.—

℞	Indian Spikenard (*Jatamansi*) . . .	2	drams.
	Water	½	pint.

Macerate for 1 hour and strain.

Dose:—2 ounces t.d.s.

Hysteria.—

℞	Asafœtida (*Hing*) . .	1	grain.
	Maschi (*Kastori*) . .	3	grains.
	Gum (*Gond*) . . .	30	grains.
	Cinnamon water . .	1½	ounces.

Hysterical Fits.—

℞	Aloes (*Musabar*) . .	20	grains.
	Asafœtida (*Hing*) . .	20	grains.
	Honey, *q.s.* for a pill mass.		

Divide into 12 pills.

Dose :—1 pill b.d.s.

Influenza Pill.—

℞	Ginger (*Sonth*) .	equal parts —5 grains.
	Asafœtida (*Hing*) .	
	Liquorice (*Mulathi*) .	
	Gum (*Babul*) . .	

Dose :—1 pill t.d.s.

Influenza Cough.—

℞	Ginger (*Sonth*) . .	5	grains.
	Long pepper (*Pipul*) .	5	grains.
	Kakra Singhi . . .	15	grains.

Dose :—1 powder three times a day.

Influenza Infusion.—

℞	Cinnamon . .	1	teaspoonful.
	Cloves (powdered) .	5	cloves.
	Ginger (powdered) .	½	teaspoonful.

Add 1 seer water.

Boil for 15 minutes. A very good remedy.

Dose :—1 ounce t.d.s.

Influenza Linctus.—

℞	Atis	5	grains.
	Pipul	5	grains.
	Kakra Singhi . . .	10	grains.
	Honey or syrup . .	1	dram.

Dose:—1 dram as required.

Indigestion Pill.—

℞	Aloes (*Musabar*) . .	2	grains.
	Ginger (*Sonth*) . .	2	grains.
	Soap, *q.s.* for one pill.		

Dose :—1 pill before food.

Indigestion Powder.—

℞	Charcoal (*Koylah*) . .	5	grains.
	Ginger (*Sonth*) . . .	5	grains.
	Rhubarb	2	grains.

Dose:—1 powder after food.

For Indigestion.—

℞	Ginger (*Sonth*) . .	5	grains.
	Bicarbonate of soda . .	15	grains.
	Infus. Cloves . . .	1	ounce.

A carminative and antacid.

For Indigestion.—

℞	Ginger (*Sonth*) . . .	2 drams.
	Brandy	4 ounces.
	Leave for 4 days.	
	Add syrup . . .	6 ounces.

Dose:—2 or 3 teaspoonfuls.

Influenza Powder (Expectorant).—

℞	Long Pepper (*Pipul*) .	equal parts —3 drams.
	Ginger (*Sonth*) .	
	Cinnamon (*Dalchini*) .	
	Caraway (*Jira*) .	
	Pepper (*Kala mirch*) .	

Dose:—½ to 1 dram t.d.s.

Insomnia.—

℞	Camphor (*Kapur*) . .	3 grains.
	Asafœtida (*Hing*) . .	3 grains.

Dose:—1 pill b.d.s.

For Itching of Skin.—

℞	Lime water . . .	*āā* 2 ounces.
	Glycerine . . .	
	Water . . .	

Laxative.—

℞	Senna leaves . . .	1 ounce.
	Ginger (*Sonth*) . . .	30 grains.
	Cloves (*Long*) . . .	30 grains.
	Water (boiling) . .	10 ounces.

Allow to stand for 1 hour and strain.

Laxative.—

℞	Tamarind fruit (*Imli*)	1	ounce.
	Dates (*Chuhara*)	1	ounce.
	Milk	1	pint.

Boil and strain.

Laxative for Piles.—

℞	Ext. liquorice	2	drams.
	Senna leaves (powdered)	1	ounce.
	Coriander powder	4	drams.
	Tamarind pulp	2	ounces.
	Alu bokara	1	ounce.
	Sugar	6	ounces.

Make a confection.

Dose :—1 dram.

Laxative.—

℞	Coriander seed (powdered)	4	drams.
	Senna leaves (powdered)	10	drams.
	Tamarind pulp	12	drams.
	Cassia pulp	12	drams.
	Prunes	8	drams.
	Sugar	40	drams.
	Water	100	drams.

Dose :—1 to 2 teaspoonfuls, a safe and gentle laxative.

Laxative Powder.—

℞	Myrobalans (*Har*)	1	dram.
	Fennel fruit (*Bari sonf*)	½	dram.
	Sugar	½	dram.

Laxative Powder.—

℞	Pulv. senna leaves	10	grains.
	Liquorice (*Mulathi*)	10	grains.
	Sulphur (*Gunduk*)	5	grains.
	Caraway (*Jira*)	5	grains.

Dose:—1 powder.

Lemonade.—

℞	Limes (sliced)	5	
	Boiling water	1	pint.

Allow to cool, strain and add sugar.

A cooling drink.

For Lepric Spots.—

℞	Chaulmoogra oil	2	ounces.
	Nim oil	2	ounces.

For Lepric Ulcers.—

℞	Chaulmoogra oil	1	dram.
	Ung: simplex	1	ounce.

Leprosy.—

℞	Chaulmoogra oil . . .	5	drops.
	Cod-liver oil . . .	30	drops.

Dose:—Twice daily after food.

Leucorrhœa.—

℞	Nitre (*Shora*) . . .	10	grains.
	Alum (*Phitkari*) . . .	5	grains.
	Water	1	ounce.

For one dose t.d.s.

Leucorrhœa (Astringent) Injection.—

℞	Pomegranate fruit rind .	3	ounces.
	Cloves	2	drams.
	Water	2	pints.

Boil for 15 minutes and add alum 2 drams.

As an injection.

Leucorrhœa Injection.—

℞	Alum (*Phitkari*) . . .	1	dram.
	Zinc. sulph. (*Kasis*) . .	30	grains.
	Water	1	pint.

For Liver (Congested).—

℞	Ammon. chlor. (*Nausader*)	10	grains.
	Syrup of orange . .	2	drams.
	Infus. senna (*Sonnamakhi*)	1	ounce.

Lice.—

℞ Oil of turpentine . . ½ ounce.
Sufed damar . . . 1 dram.
Simple ointment . . 1 ounce.

Apply locally.

Lice.—

℞ Cocculus, Indian seeds
(*Kakmari bij*) . . 1 dram.
Ghee . . . . . 1 ounce.

Make a paste. Apply to skin where lice are. There should be no abraided surface.

Lumbago Liniment.—

℞ Camphor (*Kapur*) . . 1 ounce.
Sweet oil or mustard oil . 8 ounces.

For rheumatism or lumbago.

Malarial Fever Pill (Chronic).—

℞ Bonduc seed powder . 1 dram.
Mucilage, *q.s.* for a pill mass.

Divide into 12 pills.

Dose:—1 pill twice daily.

Malarial Fever Powder.—

℞	Kaladana . . .	5	grains.
	Ginger (*Sonth*) . .	5	grains.
	Black pepper (*Kala mirch*)	5	grains.
	Bonduc seed powder (*Katkalija*)	10	grains.

Dose:—Twice daily.

Malarial Fever Powder.—

℞	Kaladana . . .	20	grains.
	Black pepper . . .	5	grains.
	Atis	15	grains.

Dose:—1 powder twice daily.

Mouth (Ulcers of).—

℞	Cupri sulph. (*Tutiya*) .	5	grains.
	Honey	1	ounce.

Apply to ulcer with finger.

Mouth Wash.—

℞	Borax (*Sohaga*) . .	1	ounce.
	Glycerine . . .	5	ounces.
	Water	5	ounces.

For ulcer in mouth.

Mouth Wash.—

℞	Glycerine of borax . .	4	drams.
	Peppermint water . .	6	ounces.

Nasal Catarrh.—

℞	Boracis (*Sohaga*) .	. 10	grains.
	Common salt (*Nimak*)	. 10	grains.
	Water . . .	. 8	ounces.

For sniffing up nose.

Nipples (Sore).—

℞	Borax (*Sohaga*) .	. 1	dram.
	Simple ointment .	. 1	ounce.

Omum Water.—

℞	Ajowan seeds . .	. 1½	pounds.
	Water . . .	. 3	quarts.

Distil for 4 hours.

Dose:—1 ounce of distil.

For spasmodic colic.

Pharyngitis.—

℞	Alum (*Phitkari*) .	. 30	grains.
	Honey . . .	. 1	ounce.
	Decoction galls .	. 8	ounces.

Pharyngitis (Chronic).—

℞	Alum (*Phitkari*) .	. 1	dram.
	Water . . .	. 6	ounces.

As a gargle.

Pharyngitis (Gargle).—

℞	Bruised rind of pomegranate	2	ounces.
	Cloves	1	dram.
	Water	1	pint.

Boil for 15 minutes and add alum 1 dram.

As a gargle.

Piles.—

℞	Babul bark (bruised) .	1½	ounces.
	Water	1	pint.

Boil for 10 minutes and strain.

An astringent injection.

Piles.—

℞	Opium (*Afim*) . .	30	grains.
	Galls (*Maiphul*) . .	1	dram.
	Simple ointment . .	1	ounce.

Piles (Painful).—

℞	Rasaut	1	grain.
	Kernel of nim seed .	3	grains.
	Raisins (*Manaka*) . .	10	grains.

Dose:—2 pills at bed time.

Piles (Painful).—

℞	Black pepper (*Kala mirch*)	1	dram.
	Caraway seeds (powdered)	2	drams.
	Honey	1	ounce.

Rub up in a mortar.

Dose:—1 teaspoonful t.d.s.

Piles (Painful).—

℞		
℞	Turmeric . . .	½ ounce.
	Ganja leaves . . .	1 ounce.
	Linseed oil, *q.s.* for a paste.	

For local application.

Piles Powder.—

℞		
℞	Black pepper (*Kala mirch*)	5 grains.
	Sulphur (*Gunduk*) . .	10 grains.

Dose:—1 powder twice daily.

Piles Powder.—

℞		
℞	Sulphur (*Gunduk*) . .	10 grains.
	Acid tart. of potash .	10 grains.

Dose:—1 powder every night.

Piles Powder.—

℞		
℞	Kaladana . . .	15 grains.
	Sulphur	15 grains.

Dose:—1 powder every night.

Piles Ointment.—

℞		
℞	Galls (*Maiphul*) . .	2 drams.
	Opium	½ dram.
	Simple ointment . .	1 ounce.

Apply locally.

Piles (Confection).—

Black pepper (*Kala mirch*)	½	dram.
Caraway (*Jira*) . .	1	dram.
Sugar	3	drams.
Confection of senna .	3	drams.

Dose:—1 teaspoonful for piles.

Piles (Prolapsed and Bleeding).—

℞ Alum (*Phitkari*) . .	1	dram.
Water	1	pint.

Apply on a cloth for 15 *minutes, twice daily.*

Piles (Prolapsed and Bleeding).—

℞ Sulphate of iron . .	6	grains.
Water	2	ounces.

As an enema.

Piles with Constipation.—

℞ Chubelic myrobalans (*Har*)	1	dram.
Beleric myrobalans (*Bahera*)	1	dram.
Embelic myrobalans (*Anwala*)	1	dram.
Aniseed (*Sonf*) . .	1	dram.
Ginger (*Sonth*) . .	1	dram.
Senna leaves (*Salsa*) .	½	dram.
Black salt (*Kala nimak*) .	½	dram.

Pulverize and mix.

Dose:—1 dram in hot milk at bed time.

Prickly-heat Lotion.—

℞	Sulphate of copper . .	1 dram.
	Rose water . . .	6 ounces.

Apply daily.

Prickly-heat Powder.

℞	Camphor (*Kapur*) . .	2 grains.
	Oxide zinc . .	equal parts —2 drams.
	Boracis . . .	
	Starch . . .	

A very good remedy.

Prolapsed Anus.—

℞	Alum powder (*Phitkari*) .	2 drams.
	Water	10 ounces.

Bathe the part and reduce it.

Prolapse of Anus and Painful Piles.—

℞	Gall powder . . .	1 ounce.
	Hot water . . .	1 pint.

Boil for 10 minutes.

Use when cold. Apply locally.

Pruritus Vulvæ.—

℞	Borax (*Sohaga*) . .	4 drams.
	Camphor water . .	8 ounces.

Apply locally.

Purgative.—

℞	Myrobalans (*Har*) .	6	drams.
	Rhubarb (*Revanchini*) .	1	dram.
	Water	4	ounces.

Boil for 10 minutes.

Dose:—The whole for one dose.

Purgative.—

℞	Myrobalans (*Chhoti har*) .	6	drams.
	Cinnamon powder (*Dalchini*)	1	dram.
	Water	4	ounces.

Boil for 10 minutes.

Drink when cold.

Purgative.—

℞	Kaladana (powdered) .	1	ounce.
	Rock salt (*Sendha nimak*) .	1	ounce.
	Ginger (*Sonth*) . . .	1	dram.

Dose:—1 dram in milk.

Purgative.—

℞	Aloes (powdered) . .	30	grains.
	Syrup	1	ounce.

Dose:—1 teaspoonful t.d.s. till moved.

Purgative (Strong).—

℞ White turpeth (*Pithori*) . 30 grains.
Ginger (*Sonth*) . . 10 grains.
Gamboge . . . 1 grain.

Purgative Powder (Strong).—

℞ Kaladana . . . 1 dram.
Gamboge . . . 1 grain.
Ginger . . . . 10 grains.

Dose:—1 powder at once.

Rheumatism.—

℞ Lemon grass oil (*Akya ghas tel*) . . . 1 ounce.
Linseed oil (*Ulsi tel*) . 1 ounce.

For application, b.d.s.

Rheumatism.—

℞ Sulphur (*Gunduk*) . . 3 grains.
Mustard (*Rai*) . . 3 grains.
Pot. nit. (*Shora*) . . 5 grains.
Rhubarb root . . 5 grains.
Honey or sugar . . 1 ounce.

Make into a paste.

Dose:—1 teaspoonful.

Rheumatism (Chronic).—

℞	Sulphur	2	ounces.
	Nim oil	1	pint.

Rub well into the joint.

Rheumatic Joints.—

℞	Ginger (*Sonth*) (bruised) .	1	dram.
	Jaiphal (*Nutmeg*) . .	2	drams.
	Sweet oil . . .	16	ounces.

A liniment.

Rheumatic Joints.—

℞	Camphor (*Kapur*) . .	1	ounce.
	Sweet oil (*Metha tel*) .	8	ounces.

A liniment.

Rheumatic Joints.—

℞	Camphor (*Kapur*) . .	½	ounce.
	Mustard oil (*Rai-ki-tel*) .	8	ounces.

Rheumatic Liniment.—

℞	Camphor . . .	1	ounce.
	Oil of turpentine . .	8	ounces.
	Soap water, *q.s.*		

For a liniment.

Rheumatism (Muscular and Chronic).—

℞	Ammon. chlor. (*Nausader*)	15	grains.
	Infus. hemidesmus (*Salsa*)	1	ounce.

Dose:—1 ounce b.d.s.

Rheumatism and Lumbago.—

℞	Camphor (*Kapur*) . .	1	ounce.
	Linseed oil (*Ulsi tel*) .	4	ounces.

A liniment.

Rheumatism (Painful) and Lumbago.—

℞	Camphor (*Kapur*) . .	3	grains.
	Opium (*Afim*) . .	½	grain.

At bed time occasionally.

Rheumatic Powder.—

℞	Sulphur sublimate . .	10	grains.
	Sodæ bicarb. . . .	10	grains.
	Powdered colchicum .	1	grain.

Dose:—1 powder twice daily.

Ring-worm.—

℞	Kamala	2	drams.
	Linseed oil (*Ulsi tel*) .	2	ounces.

Warm and stir.

Apply when cold.

Ring-worm.—

℞	Sulphate of copper . .	20	grains.
	Galls powder . . .	1	dram.
	Simple ointment . .	1	ounce.

Rub well in daily.

Ring-worm.—

℞	Boracis (*Sohaga*) . .	2	drams.
	Vinegar (*Sirka*) . .	2	ounces.

Ring-worm.—

℞ Cassia leaves (*Dadmurdan*) 2 ounces.
Linseed oil (*Ulsi tel*), *q.s.* for a paste.

Bruise into a paste.

Scabies.—

℞	Sulphur	2	drams.
	Pot. bicarb. . . .	1	dram.
	Simple ointment . .	1	ounce.

Apply externally.

Scabies.—

℞	Sulphur (*Gunduk*) . .	2	drams.
	Kamala	4	drams.

Dust the affected parts.

Scabies.—

℞	Sulphur	1 dram.
	Til oil	1 ounce.

For local use.

Scurvy.—

℞	Juice of lime (*Nimbu*)	4 drams.
	Infus. chiretta . . .	1 ounce.

Three times a day.

Simple Ointment.—

℞	Linseed oil (*Ulsi tel*) .	8 chittacks.
	Suet (*Charbi*) . . .	8 chittacks.
	Wax	2 chittacks.

A basis for all ointments.

Soothing Drinks.—

Gruel (*Atta water*).
Arrowroot and milk.
Barley water.
Albumin water (white of one egg to a tumbler of cold water).
Linseed tea (*Ulsi pani*).
Olive oil.
Milk and water.
Milk and soda water.

Spermatorrhœa.—

℞	Camphor . . .	2	grains.
	Pil. opii . .	$\frac{1}{4}$ to $\frac{1}{2}$	grain.

Spermatorrhœa.—

℞	Camphor (*Kapur*) . .	4	grains.
	Ext. hyoscyamus . .	2	grains.

Dose:—1 pill twice daily.

Spleen Powder.—

℞	Ginger (*Sonth*) . .	10	grains.
	Rhubarb (*Ravenchini*) .	5	grains.
	Ferri sulph. (*Kasis*) .	2	grains.
	Quinine	2	grains.

Dose:—1 powder twice daily after food.

Stomatitis and Spongy Gums.—

℞	Fresh lime juice . .	1	ounce.
	Water	1	ounce.

For a mouth wash.

Synovitis (Inflamed or Bruised Joints).—

℞	Pot. nit. (*Shora*) . .	1	ounce.
	Ammon. chlor. (*Nausader*)	1	ounce.
	Water	1	pint.

Apply with cloth.

Synovitis (Painful Joint).—

℞ Aloes (*Musabar*) . .	4	drams.
Opium (*Afim*) . .	4	drams.
Rum	2	ounces.

Warm down to a paste.

Apply to joint.

Tape-worm.

℞ Root bark of pomegranate (fresh)	2	ounces.
Water	2	pints.

Boil down to 1 pint.

Dose:—2 ounces in morning, fasting. Repeat every half hour, for 4 doses. Then a dose of castor oil.

A very good remedy.

Tape-worm.

℞ Powdered butea seeds (*Palas bij*) . .	equal parts —5 grains.
Embelia ribes (*Baberung*)	
Kamala . . .	
Turpeth root (*Pithori*)	

Honey or treacle, *q.s.* for one dose.

Testicles (when Swollen).—

℞	Ammon. chlor. (*Nausader*)	1	dram.
	Methylated spirit . .	1	ounce.
	Water	6	ounces.

Apply on cloth, or lint.

Throat (Ulcers of).—

℞	Glycerine of Borax (p. 39)	equal parts.
	Cinnamon water .	

For painting throat or gargle.

Thrush.—

℞	Borax (*Sohaga*) . .	1	dram.
	Honey	1	ounce.

Apply inside of the mouth with cloth.

Tonic.—

℞	Sarsaparilla root (*Anantamul*) (bruised) . . .	1	ounce.
	Water	½	pint.

Boil for 1 hour and strain. Add sugar.

Dose:—2 ounces b.d.s.

Tonic.—

℞	Sulphate of iron . .	4	grains.
	Omum water . . .	3	ounces.
	Infus. chiretta . . .	3	ounces.

Dose:—1 ounce b.d.s.

Tonic.—

℞	Ferri sulph. (*Kasis*) . . .	2	grains.
	Infus. chiretta . . .	1	ounce.

Dose:—Twice daily.

Tonic.—

℞	Quinine	30	grains.
	Lime juice . . .	1	dram.
	Infus. cloves . . .	2	ounces.

Dose:—1 teaspoonful before meals.

Tonic.—

℞	Satgilo powder (p. 76) .	10	grains.
	Atis powder . . .	10	grains.
	Bonduc-nut powder . .	10	grains.

Dose:—1 powder twice daily.

Tonic (Bitter).—

℞	Chiretta (bruised) .	1	ounce.
	Cloves (*Long*) . .	1	teaspoonful.
	Hot water . .	1	pint.

Infuse for 6 hours.

Dose:—2 ounces twice daily.

Tonic (Bitter).—

℞	Acorus root (*Bach*) infusion . . .	1	ounce.
	Chiretta infusion . .	1	ounce.

Dose:—1 ounce b.d.s.

Tonic (Bitter).—

℞	Gulancha stem (bruised) .	1	ounce.
	Cold water . . .	1	pint.

Macerate for 1 hour and strain.

Dose:—2 ounces b.d.s.

Tonic (Iron).—

℞	Ferri sulph. (*Kasis*) . .	4	grains.
	Syrup of orange . .	2	drams.
	Infus. chiretta . . .	1	ounce.

For one dose.

Tonic (for Convalescence).—

℞	Nim bark (inner layer) .	2	ounces.
	Cloves (powdered) . .	1	dram.
	Water	1½	pints.

Boil for ¼ hour and strain.

Dose:—1 ounce t.d.s.

Tonic Pill.—

℞	Ferri sulph. (*Kasis*) . .	24	grains.
	Aloes (*Musabar*) . .	24	grains.
	Cinnamon powder . .	1	dram.
	Honey, *q.s.* for a pill mass.		

Divide into 24 pills.

Dose:—2 pills twice daily.

Tonic Powder.—

℞	Ammon. carb.	1 grain.
	Sodæ bicarb.	1 grain.
	Cinchona febrifuge	2 grains.

Dose:—1 powder once daily.

Tonic Powder.—

℞	Bonduc-nut (*Katkalija*)	5 grains.
	Black pepper	5 grains.

Dose:—Twice daily.

A good tonic.

Tonsillitis.—

℞	Alum	2 drams.
	Sugar	1 dram.
	Decoction galls	1 pint.

As a gargle.

Tooth-Powder.—

℞	Chalk (*Chuna*)	2 drams.
	Alum (*Phitkari*)	2 drams.
	Camphor (*Kapur*)	½ dram.
	Myrrh (*Bol*)	½ dram.

Tootn-Powder.—

℞	Borax (*Sohaga*)	1 dram.
	Alum (*Phitkari*)	1 dram.
	Black pepper (*Kala mirch*)	10 grains.
	Chalk (*Chuna*)	2 drams.

Tooth-Powder.—

℞	Alum (*Phitkari*) . .	}	1 dram of each.
	Gall-nut (*Maiphul*) . .		
	Sulphate of iron (*Kasis*) .		
	Catechu (*Katha*) . .		
	Chalk (*Chuna*) . .		

Tooth-Powder.—

℞	Catechu (*Katha*) . .	2 drams.
	Myrrh (*Bol*) . . .	1 dram.
	Chalk (*Karimutti*) . .	4 drams.
	Oil of cloves . . .	3 drops.

A good tooth-powder.

Tooth-Powder.—

℞	Chalk (*Chuna*) .	}	equal parts.
	Camphor (*Kapur*) .		
	Charcoal (*Koylah*) .		
	Salt (*Nimak*) . .		

Tympanites (Flatulency).—

℞	Asafœtida . . .	30 grains.
	Water	6 ounces.

For an enema.

Ulcers.—

℞	Oxide zinc . . .	2	drams.
	Pot. bicarb. . . .	1	dram.
	Simple ointment . .	1	ounce.

An astringent ointment.

Ulcers.—

℞	Oil of turpentine . .	1	ounce.
	Piney (*Sufed damar*) .	1	dram.
	Wax	4	drams.
	Lard	4	drams.

Heat gently and stir while cooling.

Turpentine ointment.

Ulcers (Chronic).—

℞	Catechu (*Katha*) . .	1	dram.
	Wax	2	drams.
	Honey	4	drams.

An ointment.

Ulcers (Chronic Watery).—

℞	Myrobalans (powdered) .	1	dram.
	Catechu (*Katha*) . .	1	dram.
	Simple ointment . .	1	ounce.

An ointment.

Ulcers (Indolent).—

℞	Capsicum (*Lal mirch*) (powdered)	1	dram.
	Simple ointment	1	ounce.

Ulcers on Penis.—

℞	Alum	20	grains.
	Water	1	ounce.

For local application.

Ulcers (Sloughing).—

℞	Borax (*Sohaga*)	2	drams.
	Camphor water	1	pint.

As a dressing.

Ulcers (in Mouth).—

℞	Borax (*Sohaga*)	1	ounce.
	Glycerine	5	ounces.
	Water	6	ounces.

Uterine Hæmorrhage.—

℞	Asoka bark	4	ounces.
	Water	1	pint.

Boil down to a quarter and strain.

Dose :—1 ounce t.d.s.

Vomiting (of Cholera).—

℞ Lemon grass oil (*Agya ghas tel*) . . . . . 5 drops.

In ½ teaspoonful of sugar.

Worm (Round-worm) Powder.—

℞ Asafœtida (*Hing*) . . . 4 grains.
Chiretta powder . . . 10 grains.

Dose:—1 every night.

Worms (Thread).—

℞ Salt (*Nimak*) . . . . ½ dram.
Warm water . . . . 6 ounces.

Inject into back passage.

Chief drugs for dispensary use, which should be stocked in wide-mouthed 4-oz. bottles.

For dispensary work, the following stock of bazaar drugs should always be kept in wide-mouthed bottles for the making of stock powders, pills, liniments, aquæ, and any prescription which comes in :-

Ajowan seeds.
Alum.
Ammon. chlor.
Anwala.
Asafœtida.
Atis.
Babul gum.
Bonduc-nut.
Borax.
Camphor.
Capsicum.
Caraway seeds.
Cardamom.
Catechu.
Chuna (*Lime*).
Cinnamon powder.
Common salt.
Copper sulph.
Coriander seed.
Cubebs.
Dill seeds.
Gall powder.
Ginger.
Har (*Myrobalans*).
Hindi salsa.
Isaphgul.
Kakra singhi.
Kaladana powder.
Kamala powder.
Kurchi seeds.
Liquorice.
Moringa oil.
Nutmeg.
Pepper.
Pipul.
Pot. nit.
Rock salt.
Sulphate of iron.
Sulphur.
Sugar.
Turpentine oil.

Stock powders, pills, aquæ, etc., for dispensary use.

The following stock powders, pills, aquæ, and liniments should be kept ready made up for issue to out-patients :—

Aquæ, etc.

(from Bazaar Medicines).

CHAPTER IV.

Stock medicines for emergencies and first aid.

It is advisable in every dispensary to keep a first-aid case or medicine chest ready for taking out to emergencies. Good medicine chests and cases with two or three drawers and a compartment for bottles can now be purchased from any good surgical instrument maker. They are either of tin (the compartments being one on top of the other are joined by side pieces when pulled up) or of leather with two drawers and a compartment for bottles beneath. It is not difficult to get a local carpenter to make a small case with three small drawers which can be used as an emergency case. Size is generally $10\frac{1}{2} \times 6\frac{1}{2}$, and depth according to the number of drawers.

The contents of each drawer is here suggested.

Top drawer.—Size $10 \times 6 \times 2$ deep chiefly for pills and powders in small boxes as follows:—

Pot. Permang. crystals (for snake-bite and antiseptic lotion) 2 drams.

Cholera pills (*see* Index).

Boracic powder—For lotion for sore eyes (*see* Index).

Laxative powder (*see* Index).

Opium pills—For pain, shock and diarrhœa.

Colic pills (*see* Index).

Diarrhœa powder (*see* Index).

Second drawer for surgical necessaries.—
Same size.

Packet of lint.

Packet of gauze.

Packet of cotton-wool.

Two or three 2-inch bandages.

Surgical needles in small box.

Two artery forceps (one for needle holder).

Surgical scissors.

Scalpel or surgical knife.

Small reel of sterilized silk No. 0 size in methylated spirits.

Third and bottom compartment.—
Size $6 \times 10 \times 4\frac{3}{4}$ deep.

To hold a small rack for holding six or eight bottles which can be drawn out (bottles standing upright). Size of bottles about 2 oz.

The following contents suggested :—

Tinct. opii—For pain and colic.

Castor oil—For intestinal disturbance and eye drops.

Linseed oil—For scalds and mild burns.

Tinct. iodine—For painting wounds.

Methylated spirits—For sterilizing needles and threads.

Tinct. ginger—For flatulency.

This compartment can conveniently have a division down the centre. One half for rack with medicines and one for hypodermic syringes, vaccines and serum. Messrs. Allen & Hanbury make a very good emergency case on these lines.

INDEX.